Ulcerative Colitis
NOT
for
Life

Caro Beth

Ulcerative Colitis
NOT
for
Life

A Healing Journey
from
Overwhelmed
to
Self-Empowered

Ulcerative Colitis NOT for Life
Paperback Edition 2023
Copyright © 2023 by Caro Beth
ISBN: 9798390730393

The information in this book is not intended as medical advice and cannot replace the consultation with a competent physician. All content is for educational and informational purposes only. Any recommendations should be implemented only under the direct advice of a competent and qualified therapist and are at the user's responsibility and risk.

This narration is subjective and represents the author's personal experience. All names occurring in this book are entirely fictitious.

For readability reasons, only the masculine form is used in some places and refers to both genders.

About the Author

Caro Beth, MA, qualified as a certified Food Matters Institute nutrition coach in 2023. She is also an independent documentary filmmaker and translator.

After her son was diagnosed with ulcerative colitis in 2016, supporting him on his healing journey became her priority. Her intensive research into the causes of chronic inflammatory bowel disease (IBD) and her search for natural therapy options led her to the Specific Carbohydrate Diet (SCD) and the GAPS Diet. Both diets enabled her son to reverse his disease and live with no medication and no IBD symptoms today.

As a nutrition coach specialising in gut health and the SCD, Caro Beth assists patients with IBD and other gut conditions with their dietary, lifestyle, and behaviour changes. With her books, she intends to give patients hope and courage and to support them with their natural approach to curing their illnesses.

Caro Beth is German and lives in Ireland.

Visit her website on mygutsense.com
Facebook: Caro Beth - Author

I dedicate this book to my son.
Our children can reveal our worst, but also our best, qualities.
My son and his colitis have brought out the best in me.

*"So now faith, hope and love abide,
These three, but the greatest of these is love."*
(1 Corinthians 13:13)

CONTENTS

Introduction

Sometimes our children need us most when we expect them to eventually go their ways and give us more space to follow our interests. That is the experience I had when my sixteen-year-old son Luca was diagnosed with ulcerative colitis, and I was attempting to return to my professional career. Luca's severe illness not only threw me entirely off track concerning my personal goals but also brought me to my psychological and emotional limits. It was not even the illness that troubled me so much but the pessimistic prognoses of representatives of mainstream medicine and the feelings of hopelessness and fear they evoked.

Initially, I believed any information that conventional doctors and the pharmaceutical industry are spreading about the alleged incurability of ulcerative colitis. I was convinced it was confirmed that no other options were available for patients than a lifetime use of medication correlating with substantial side effects. I could already see the development of my son's disease in front of my inner eye – a downward spiral connected with a lot of suffering, possibly ending with the surgical removal of his colon and an artificial bowel outlet. But what if all of this was not true, and if there was another way than that of the medical establishment?

Today, the fact that I had come across Elaine Gottschall's website on the internet and had learned about the Specific Carbohydrate Diet (SCD) appears to me as providence. Elaine Gottschall was a biochemist, cell biologist, and highly devoted mother. In the 1950s, the SCD saved Gottschall's eight-year-old daughter Judy, who had severe ulcerative colitis, from the removal of her colon. This elimination diet was developed by the New Yorker paediatrician Dr Sidney V. Haas. He was the fifteenth doctor whom the Gottschalls consulted with their severely ill child, and he was the first one who asked about Judy's diet. The Gottschalls changed their daughter's diet according to the SCD, and Judy's healing could begin.

Thousands of patients with inflammatory bowel disease and other gut conditions were able to gain back their health with the help of the SCD. However, mainstream doctors still do not acknowledge the role that diet plays in the genesis and treatment of these diseases. That is *one* reason patients are usually not offered this dietary intervention as a treatment option. That the pharmaceutical industry cannot exploit it certainly is another reason.

When Luca and I decided to try the SCD and take his treatment into our own hands, I made his recovery the priority in my life. It lasted over a year until his colitis symptoms (frequent diarrhoea with mucus and blood and severe pain during flare-ups) disappeared. We stopped Luca's prescribed medications a few months after his diagnosis because they had been ineffective and had led to numerous adverse effects.

Luca's healing journey was strenuous, and many relapses made us doubtful about the efficacy of our treatment method. In addition, Luca suffered from a contamination phobia, making it even harder for him to heal. Nevertheless, we did not give up hope and kept going. Luca's illness became the biggest challenge in my whole life, but I was able to use it as a chance for my inner growth. For Luca, his healing journey was also connected with an enormous inner maturing process.

Luca has been without any symptoms since 2017 and is in good health. Nutrition, according to the SCD and the GAPS Diet, respectively, has become normal for him. His health is my greatest gift and makes me grateful and happy every day. I have learned what it means to love a person unconditionally, and maybe unconditional love is the most effective medicine of all.

Our healing success and that of numerous other patients show that there is an alternative to the conventional approach, which consists of medication and is only symptomatic. The effectiveness of the SCD as a treatment method for inflammatory bowel disease could be verified in various scientific studies. In the USA, it is used in some clinics to treat patients with Crohn's disease and ulcerative colitis. One of the leading children's clinics, the Seattle Children's Hospital, is leading the way to the future.

Hopefully, this paradigm shift, which is taking place in the USA, will also influence the mainstream therapy for inflammatory bowel disease elsewhere. However, at present, patients can count themselves lucky if they come across the SCD and attempt to reverse their illness.

With this personal experience report, I intend to give fate a helping hand and support patients on their journey back to health.

Background

Only about 50 years ago, chronic inflammatory bowel disease (IBD) was still considered a rare condition. Nowadays, especially in the highly industrialised Western world, more and more people are affected, and the number is rising. According to the Centers for Disease Control and Prevention (CDC), about 3.1 million adults (1.3 per cent) in the US have been diagnosed with IBD, which includes Crohn's disease and ulcerative colitis. *(1)*

In Ireland, at least 40,000 people are affected by these conditions. According to Prof. Glen Doherty, Consultant Gastroenterologist at St. Vincent's University Hospital, Dublin, the number of new cases diagnosed with IBD each year has tripled from 2010 to 2020. In 2020 it was estimated that 0.5 per cent of the population suffered from ulcerative colitis and 0.3 per cent from Crohn's disease. *(2)*

The patient's general health and quality of life suffer tremendously under these grave and debilitating conditions, usually accompanied by deficiency symptoms and weight loss. Patients feel weak and miserable and can also be affected by depression. Often they cannot participate in social life or cope with their working day. All of this is especially tragic because inflammatory bowel disease tends to occur for the first time between the age of 16 and 24.

Chronic inflammatory bowel disease proceeds in phases. During an active phase or flare-up of ulcerative colitis, patients suffer from frequent diarrhoea with mucus and blood accompanied by abdominal cramps and pain. Some patients lose so much blood during flare-ups that they need blood transfusions regularly. During remission, inflammation subsides, and symptoms are not as severe or don't occur at all.

One aim of IBD therapy is to prolong the remission phase as much as possible. For this purpose, doctors usually prescribe mesalazine. In some cases, additional anti-inflammatory medications such as cortisone or immunosuppressive drugs are prescribed during a flare-up to suppress the symptoms and the immune system.

From an orthodox medical view, ulcerative colitis is regarded as a chronic and incurable condition. In the genesis of the disease, the role of genetic factors is emphasised. Most patients have to take medications for the rest of their lives, and as it is common for their symptoms to get worse over time, it is necessary to change over to stronger medications or different groups of drugs. However, this can result in even more severe adverse reactions. Above all, representatives of conventional medicine claim that ulcerative colitis can only be cured by the complete surgical removal of the colon. This operation is accompanied by the creation of an artificial bowel outlet (stoma) and the social stigma attached to it.

Although allopathic drugs have their justification, they should not be taken over more extended periods because of their side effects. In addition, these drugs only manage symptoms while not dealing with their root causes. Therefore it is recommendable that patients look for alternatives to treat their condition.

Unfortunately, most mainstream doctors still claim that a patient's nutrition and lifestyle do not impact the disease development. However, scientific studies and the personal experience of numerous patients prove the opposite.

A Time of Uncertainty

You come in,
And the sun goes up.
I love you,
To the moon and back.
You are everything to me,
You fill my life with joy.

February 2017
I am looking at the framed photograph of Luca standing next to me on my bedside table. He was four months old then. His big blue eyes are focused on me, open and full of confidence – a glance only a baby can have. I remember when he opened his eyes for the first time after birth and looked at me extensively. "Oh, this is what you look like," he appeared to say. A window to his soul had opened for me, and I felt my eyes moist with tears.

Recently, I often look at this photo. I can't escape this gaze. Sometimes I cannot suppress my tears. These open and innocent eyes, the huge responsibility I feel upon me and the boundless love I have for my son. Have I done all the right things? Could I have prevented him from getting his disease? Today Luca is 16 ½ years old. For three months now, we have known that he has ulcerative colitis.

It all began last summer. However, the disease had started developing much earlier. Nobody can tell exactly when. We flew to Frankfurt to visit my mother at the end of June. Luca had been looking forward to our holidays for a long time. It meant six weeks of playing football with his friends in summery weather. He also had ideas for new football videos that he would film with his action camera and upload on his YouTube channel.

The only thing he did not like regarding our holiday plans was the long journey from the Northwest of Ireland to the small Hessian town in the Rhine-Main-Area where I had grown up. Luca was particularly worried about the flight as he is terrified of flying or, rather, of crashing. Therefore it did not surprise us that he had diarrhoea on the day of our departure. After breakfast, Alex − my partner and Luca's dad − drove us to Abbeytown, where we took the train to Dublin.

From Dublin Connolly Station we took the bus to the airport where we had to wait several hours. The actual flight was the shortest part of our journey. We arrived at my mother's house late in the evening, exhausted but happy and full of expectations. We had made it once again, and everything had gone well. Contented, we went to bed. The following day, we would have a sleep-in and then take it easy.

On our second day, Luca wanted to go to

the football pitch for the first time to try out his new football shoes. However, as his diarrhoea returned, he couldn't. We didn't take too much notice of it, as we believed it had to do with travelling. Luca kept eating what he usually ate. It would go away again. The only real nuisance was that Luca could not leave the house and put his plans into action. When things had not improved a few days later, I got him charcoal tablets and the common diarrhoea drug Imodium. He took both.

I noticed Luca withdrew in his room more frequently and became increasingly quiet. The reason for this became apparent when I wanted to use the bathroom. I opened the toilet lid, and everything was red. I called my mother to show her my alarming discovery. Horrified, we looked at each other. There was diarrhoea with a lot of bloody mucus in the toilet. When I had composed myself again, I went to Luca to talk to him. Finally, he could share his secret with me and no longer had to hide away with his fear.

I told him that we had to get ready to see a doctor. Before going to the group practice my mother visits, I filled a sample of Luca's bloody stool in a container. It was Friday afternoon, and I knew the practice would soon be closing for the weekend.

The doctor where we landed did not seem to be very motivated and probably only wanted to be off for the weekend. He palpated Luca's abdomen. He didn't even take a glance at Luca's stool sample. He couldn't advise me on what would be best for Luca to eat now. We were already half out of the door when he said we should come around again if Luca's diarrhoea did not improve.

Our visit to the doctor was very unsatisfactory, and we could have spared the effort. Nevertheless, his composure – in retrospect, I would call it indifference – calmed me because, seemingly, there was no reason to panic. I assumed that Luca must have caught some virus. My mother and I provided him with food that we thought was easy to digest and would not stress his gut too much. I was convinced it was only a matter of time until Luca recovered from his diarrhoea. The symptoms got slightly better at times, but he still felt groggy.

In the meantime, I started a job as a freelance translator, which I had been chasing after for weeks. Our time in Germany passed by quickly. Looking back, I wonder how I found inner peace to work. Partly this was due to my ignorance at the time. And my work also diverted me from continuously thinking about Luca's diarrhoea which had already become our main conversation topic.

As Luca's diarrhoea persisted almost a week after our first visit to the doctor, we went back there. This time, a very pleasant female doctor took care of Luca. She made sure that a blood sample was taken immediately and told us that it was crucial to perform a stool test to find out if there was blood in Luca's stool. I told her that on our last visit, I had already informed her colleague about Luca's bloody diarrhoea and had shown him a stool sample stained red. She looked at Luca's file on her computer and was surprised that her colleague had not even mentioned the large amount of blood in Luca's stool. His stool sample should have been examined much earlier, but nothing had happened so far, thanks to the doctor's negligence.

For the first time, a doctor mentioned that Luca's diarrhoea could be a sign of ulcerative colitis. At this point, I had no idea what this term meant. I looked it up at home online, and what I found out did not sound uplifting. I tried to worry as little as possible about it. After all, it was only a suspicion. I still believed that Luca had caught a rather persistent gut virus.

A few days later, we got the result of his stool test. No bacteria pointing to infection had been found, but it had been confirmed that there was blood in Luca's stool. We were advised to make an appointment for a colonoscopy, and I was relieved to get one relatively soon. Meanwhile, our return journey was coming closer. I knew it could take extremely long to get an appointment with a specialist in Ireland, so I was keen on getting the examination done in Germany.

During a preliminary surgery talk, the gastroenterologist, roughly at the end of his thirties, explained what would happen during the examination. He said we could also wait for further development for another six weeks. If it was ulcerative colitis, there were rather good options to treat this condition with medication nowadays. I asked him if there was anything that we should give attention to concerning Luca's nutrition. He answered that diet played no role in ulcerative colitis, neither in its genesis nor treatment.

"Little influences our health more than the foods we consume. The modern diet is a prescription for obesity, metabolic problems, and all kinds of other chronic diseases (1)."
(Chris Kresser, Functional Medicine expert and author of "Unconventional Medicine")

The gastroenterologist said Luca should eat what he likes. I was surprised by this answer. To my knowledge, you eliminate certain foods when you have diarrhoea to help the gut recover. However, for the moment, I accepted his opinion. I also explained that Luca had been under extreme stress for a long time and that he often reacted to stress with diarrhoea. "But stress doesn't make bloody diarrhoea," he replied. I noticed a certain arrogance in his voice and asked myself how he could be so sure of that. Today I know that his claim was not correct.

Luca's colonoscopy and ultrasound scan appointment was roughly a week after this conversation. We had been given a few packets of a powder with which we were supposed to mix a laxative. In the meantime, Luca felt a lot better. His stool was back to normal, and we couldn't see any blood in it. We had the feeling that Luca had gotten over his illness. We only wanted the colonoscopy to be on the safe side.

On the day before the examination, Luca was not allowed to eat anything after midday. After this, he had to drink three to four litres of the laxative solution divided over several hours. In the end, he could hardly get down any more of the stuff, but I encouraged him to go on, and he made it after all. During the night, the laxative started to work, and as Luca had to go to the toilet permanently, he would rather have stayed seated there.

I also hardly got any sleep. Luca was in a pitiable condition. He was exhausted, and in the previous weeks, he had lost quite some weight. It surprised me that he got over the torture of going to the toilet all night without the slightest trace of blood in his stool. The laxative must have been very aggressive, as, after this procedure, the toilet was more pristine than with any toilet cleaner.

The next morning, Luca felt very weak, didn't want to go anywhere, and only wanted to sleep. I could understand him very well as I wasn't feeling much different. Nonetheless, I tried to persuade him and told him he could make it. When this was unsuccessful, I tried to put some pressure on him, but this also didn't help. Finally, I had no choice but to ring the doctor's office and cancel the appointment.

The receptionist asked me if Luca could not come for the ultrasound scan, at least. I told her that I would try to talk him into it. In the meantime, he had locked himself in my bedroom. I doubted that we would make it to any examination at all. Now my mother also got involved. At some point, we must have gotten so much on Luca's nerves that he agreed to the ultrasound scan but nothing else. I secretly hoped he would also endure the colonoscopy once he was in the surgery.

The gastroenterologist started with the ultrasound scan. Luca could see the monitor's screen, and during the examination, the doctor named the organs that were just visible and explained that they all looked healthy. Then he announced that he would put in the tube for the sedative. Luca looked at me in terror. "Mama, you told me I only have to get the ultrasound scan!" I tried to persuade him to endure the second part of the examination – the colonoscopy – as well, but without any success.

"You got this far and got done with all of this shit. If I were in your place and had blood in my stool, I would see that I get this examination done as well," the doctor inferred. I felt powerless and hoped Luca would submit to the gastroenterologist's authority. I suggested that Luca discuss everything with the doctor again, and I would wait outside. Before I left the room, I turned around again and said: "Luca, I am not going away. I won't leave you alone." – "She couldn't do that anyway," remarked the doctor. Until today, I don't know what he wanted to say with this. He probably considered me a real hen, but why do I waste a thought about it at all?

Only a few minutes after me, Luca came into the waiting room. Relieved, he told me that we could go home now. I was speechless. I couldn't force him to do anything; it was his decision at sixteen years old. Later, he told me it hadn't been the examination he had been afraid of but the sedation. He had believed that he would get full sedation and had feared that he might not wake up again. Luca is an absolute control freak, and the thought of losing control over anything does cause him a lot of stress.

We had only a few days left of our holiday if you could call it a holiday. Luca used the remaining time to rest and build up his strength again. The European Football Championships and the Olympic Games were his only distractions. These two events allowed him to take his mind off his illness which had destroyed all his ambitious plans for our stay in Germany. It saddened him, but he didn't even complain about it. He was simply glad that his diarrhoea and the terrible fear of the blood in his stool had ended. All he wanted was to go back home again.

On our arrival in Dublin, cool and wet weather awaited us. Luca and I continued our journey by bus and train. It remained overcast and rainy. The final station was Abbeytown, where Alex was waiting for us. He took us in his arms and was thrilled to have us back again. Back home, Rover, our black Labrador mongrel, ran towards us, wagging his tail. Our tomcat Ruby commented on our return with a loud "meow". Alex had already prepared a cottage pie, and we had supper together.

I enjoyed the view of the mountain range that rises near the end of our property. In the evening sun that had found a small gap in the thick blanket of clouds, the mountains looked like a section of a miniature railway landscape. Luca and I were glad that the stressful time in Germany was behind us. It was the beginning of August. Luca had another four weeks left before school started again.

Time passed without the bloody diarrhoea reoccurring. Now we were sure that a virus had been its cause. We thought that this alarming chapter had come to an end. Luca tried to practise his football skills as much as possible to compensate for his lost time. However, his constant hunger was still a problem for him. Before he went to the football pitch, I often prepared him porridge, pancakes from wholemeal flour, or a portion of wholemeal pasta with tomato sauce. Then he would mostly take bananas, oat crackers, and a chocolate bar with him in case he needed a quick energy boost. In addition to this, for his urgent energy needs, I bought him an ample supply of dextrose energy tablets in the pharmacy.

Luca constantly feared getting hungry while being out and about because when this did happen, he felt lousy. He suffered from dizziness. His ears rang, his arms tingled, and his hands felt cold. In addition, he felt a hot and burning sensation in his abdomen, often followed by diarrhoea. We had already told Dr Morrin, our family practitioner, about this a few times, but he had not been able to put the pieces together. He didn't take Luca's symptoms seriously and told us more or less that it was all in his head.

"A doctor of the highest calibre treats an illness before it happens."
(A principle in Traditional Chinese Medicine)

A long time after this, we learnt from an Irish alternative practitioner and nutritionist that celiac disease was widely spread in Ireland. This therapist was the first one who took sufficient time to listen to Luca's story. Luca felt they fitted together and that he was in good hands.

The high incidence of celiac disease, particularly in the Northwest of Ireland, is undoubtedly related to several factors. However, this region's extreme lack of sunshine shouldn't be underestimated as an underlying cause. Vitamin D levels of the people living there are far too low, and sufficient vitamin D is crucial for proper immune function.

I don't understand why our general practitioner had not considered testing Luca for gluten sensitivity much earlier in his disease development. All of his symptoms could have suggested that he had a gluten problem. One time, Luca made the apt remark that Dr Morrin "let him run into the open knife", meaning that his doctor had not taken the necessary steps to prevent him from further damage.

Luca was suffering from a constant lack of energy. In his despair, he reached for chocolate bars, cereals, and whole packets of oat crackers more and more frequently. Once, Luca mixed a special "calorie bomb" from ice cream, peanut butter, bananas, and anything very calorie-dense to have enough energy for his training. Food that, in his view, didn't provide him with energy, he refused to eat. These foods included many types of vegetables, which Luca considered to be mainly for decorative purposes. He frequently got hungry at night and had to eat something urgently to avoid dizziness. In the mornings, the doors of the kitchen cupboards would often be wide open because he had been in search of an emergency source of energy.

I observed this rather helplessly because I couldn't put myself in his shoes. If it happens to me that I have to fast for some hours, it doesn't cause me low energy levels or dizziness. I simply couldn't understand how someone could be hungry again after eating. Although I can't remember suffering from low energy during puberty, I assumed that Luca's condition had to do with hormonal changes, his growth, and all his sports activities. I was not at all impressed with what he was eating. A healthy diet, or what I considered healthy, had always been important to me, and I always wanted Luca to develop an awareness of this as well. However, I let him get away with his unhealthy eating habits as I thought this was just a phase that would pass.

If I had been aware of the disastrous consequences of Luca's diet, I would not have accepted his poor food choices. Especially because I knew that healthy eating habits are not primarily about getting enough calories but that it is crucial to supply your body with sufficient vitamins and other vital nutrients. At this point, I also wasn't aware that Luca's gut had lost its ability to digest his food properly, which resulted in deficiency symptoms. The "hot feeling" in his tummy, which Luca interpreted as hunger, wasn't only hunger but also the result of inflammation.

A few days before the end of Luca's

holidays, I mentioned "school". It was a sensitive topic, as Luca had not been able to attend school for one and a half years. He had been plagued by diarrhoea every morning before he was supposed to go to school. As a psychologist had diagnosed him with social phobia, he had been entitled to home tuition. Luca had promised us that he would try to go back to school in the new term. We were optimistic because he had passed his written exams before the holidays. With my knowledge today, I am sure the exam stress triggered his colitis.

I bought a new school uniform for Luca, and when I came home with it, the doors of the kitchen cupboards were wide open again. The terrible, burning abdominal pain had returned, and in his despair, Luca had eaten a whole packet of cereals out of the box. Besides, the bloody diarrhoea was back. We were shocked. On no account had I wanted Luca to become ill again. I was convinced that the stress must have triggered the diarrhoea. Maybe Luca just wasn't ready to go back to school again. At this point, he didn't have anything else on his mind other than a career as a professional football player. So we decided to allow him a year without school. He was neither able nor willing to concentrate on anything else but football, and he feared he would run out of time.

I met with the school principal to familiarise him with our plans. I was worried that he would think I had lost my mind. All the more, I was surprised that it all made sense to him. "Maybe he has it in him to become a professional footballer. I can understand that you don't want to be in his way. He has to try it out. If it doesn't work out for him, at least his mind is free to go back to studying." I was astonished to hear this from a school principal. We were happy with our decision, and Luca could hardly believe his luck. He was highly motivated and went to the football pitch as often as possible. He was determined not to let anything ruin his ambitious plans. We were convinced that having the freedom to follow his personal goals would do him good and contribute to his complete recovery. Luca's health had become my priority. Anything else, including school, was secondary now. However, the bloody diarrhoea returned every two to three weeks and with it, the fear and uncertainty that Luca, Alex and I experienced.

I went to our general practitioner and asked him to refer Luca to a gastroenterologist. We regretted that Luca had avoided the colonoscopy in Germany, as it can take so long to see a specialist in Ireland. I mentioned I was afraid Luca could have ulcerative colitis after all. To get more information on this condition, I had borrowed a book about inflammatory bowel disease from the library. However, our GP said there was no blood in the stool of patients with ulcerative colitis and that he did not believe Luca was suffering from it. I was confused by his statement, as all my other information sources listed "bloody stools" as a main symptom of this disease.

Until today, I don't know if our GP just wanted us to relax or if he was misinformed. Or perhaps the symptoms, which couldn't be overlooked any longer, contradicted his firm conviction that everything was only taking place in Luca's head. I asked our doctor if the blood in Luca's stool could have anything to do with his nutrition. I told him Luca ate large amounts of oat crackers because of his permanent hunger. These were also known to calm the nerves and create relatively constant blood sugar levels. Luca mostly ate these crackers without anything else, and I imagined that too much fibre of this kind could act in the gut like sandpaper. I also pointed out to our doctor that Luca's stool, also when he did not have diarrhoea, looked like fermented sourdough.

Dr Morrin believed the oat crackers had nothing to do with the symptoms. He also let me know that Luca's blood test did not confirm that he had celiac disease. Nevertheless, we tried to reduce Luca's consumption of cereals and oat crackers. My intuition told me that anything you consume in excess couldn't be good for you. For the moment, I decided to put the specialised medical literature aside. We didn't even have a proper diagnosis yet, and I believed it was better not to get too worried.

Much later, I learnt that only the presence of alpha-gliadin antibodies in the bloodstream could be confirmed with the standard lab test for celiac disease. Alpha-gliadin, however, is only one of 62 gluten peptides to which the immune system can react with the formation of antibodies. Only 50 per cent of people with celiac disease have elevated antibodies to alpha-gliadin, although they have gluten sensitivity. *(2)* You can have a gluten problem even though your lab test was negative. So Luca may have had undiagnosed celiac disease. In this context, it is also interesting that for people with celiac disease, the risk of developing ulcerative colitis or Crohn's disease is 86 times higher than for people without this condition. *(3)*

2

Diagnosis of Ulcerative Colitis

At the end of September, we received a letter from the University Clinic in Abbeytown. Luca's colonoscopy was scheduled for the 11th of November, 2016. We were glad that our uncertainty would soon come to an end. A few days before his appointment, Luca was concerned that he could have bloody diarrhoea again when the examination was due. I tried to convince him that this would not be the case. However, the night before the examination, his fear turned into reality. The diarrhoea was back, and with it, considerable amounts of blood. Luca's fear and sadness weighed him down. I took him tightly in my arms and gently caressed his back.

On the day before the colonoscopy, he wasn't allowed to eat anything after midday. He was terrified that the next morning, he would have to wait long in the hospital without breakfast and would faint. I promised him to intervene if the waiting time got unbearable. On the following day, we let Luca sleep as long as possible. I took sufficient food with me so he would have something to eat straight after the examination. His appointment was at nine o'clock.

On the drive to Abbeytown, we hardly spoke a word. Dense drizzle was running down the screens of our old rusty Ford. It was a cold, grey morning. The few steps from the hospital car park to the clinic entrance were enough to get completely soaked. Standing a little beside myself, I was grateful when a voluntary worker approached us and helped us find our way. We registered in the Gastroenterology ward, and then we had to wait. Alex had come with us as well. Luca was rather settled. Above all else, he was sure what he wouldn't have: a sedative!

There were mostly older people in the waiting room. All the patients who returned from their examination were relatively slow and wobbly on their feet. It moved me to see how they were cared for with a cup of tea and a sandwich after the ordeal. They were not allowed to leave the clinic immediately because of the anaesthesia. Luca was determined not to stay a minute longer than what was necessary. Even if the examination were slightly unpleasant, he would reject getting a sedative. Finally, it was his turn. I accompanied him.

He had to take off all his clothes and put on a hospital green gown which was open in the back. When the nurse came in with the enema, I left the room. Shortly after this, she called me back in again. She said it would take ten minutes until Luca could empty his bowels. They were almost empty anyway because of Luca's diarrhoea during the night.

I felt infinitely sorry for Luca, lying on the bed, waiting for any bowel movements. He was looking pale and vulnerable. Had I been able to swap places with him, I wouldn't have hesitated for a second, but he had to deal with this himself. It was *his* illness. As long as we were still alone, I took Luca in my arms, hugged him tightly, and told him that he would be all right.

A knock on the door, and Dr Cody, the gastroenterologist, entered. Luca's file was attached to his clipboard. I informed him that Luca did not want to be sedated and asked Dr Cody if I could talk to him after the colonoscopy. He looked at me in bewilderment. Unfortunately, this was impossible as he had to perform one examination after another. A nurse would discuss everything with us afterwards. Then he disappeared again.

Shortly after, Luca was picked up. I looked him in the eyes. "Take care!" I said gently. Back in the waiting room, I sat down next to Alex and told him what had happened. The time we were waiting seemed like an eternity. Alex got himself a coffee. I didn't want anything. In my thoughts, I was with Luca. Whenever someone opened the waiting room door, I thought it was him. I was very tense. When he finally came in, he looked very relieved. He sat beside me and asked what I had to eat for him. I passed him the bag with the food, and he started with a banana and a few oat crackers. Then he said it had been okay; of course, the examination had not been pleasant but not painful.

The nurse asked us to come into her office.

With the help of an illustration, she explained to us that Luca had pancolitis. In plain language, his entire colon was inflamed, causing the bloody diarrhoea. Luca only wanted to know if he could perform any sport with this condition, as his goal was to become a professional football player. He was relieved when the nurse told him there were also famous and successful athletes with colitis. She passed us a prescription on which she had written the names of two medications: Asacolon and Salofalk enemas. She said Luca would have to take these for at least two years. Before we left, the nurse gave me a few information leaflets about IBD. She said I could also find her name and contact details in the brochures if I had further questions. My head felt empty. Luca wanted to take the fastest way home. On the way back, we tried to get his medication.

What I wasn't aware of then was that Luca's illness would become the biggest challenge of my life so far. The three of us were at the start of a strenuous journey on which we would learn a lot. Luca's first reaction was a relief because the examination, which had been ahead of him for so long, was over. Besides, finally, his suffering had a name, and he could put it into context. There were drugs available that would cure him. At least, this is what he thought at the time.

In the afternoon, he wanted to take the first Asacolon tablet but couldn't swallow it. It was huge, and he feared it would get stuck in his throat. I reassured him that this wouldn't happen. Although he kept trying, he couldn't manage to get it down. I found some multivitamin capsules I had never used, which were bigger than his tablets. I swallowed one of them with a glass of water to demonstrate to Luca how easy this was. He tried it again but failed. I told him that he shouldn't put himself under pressure for now. It would eventually work out for him if he tried to relax.

In the evening, I started doing my online research into ulcerative colitis. I looked up both English and German health websites. I kept finding information that was congruent in terms of content and that represented the mainstream medical view. The authors stated that the cause of the disease was unknown. However, they assumed an abnormal immunological reaction against the gut flora was responsible. Ulcerative colitis is classified as an autoimmune disease and is supposed to be chronic and incurable.

As if all of this had not been enough to give me an enormous shock, I also learnt that most patients' symptoms worsen over time. As a result, these patients require therapy with corticosteroids. And if this does not show the expected results, it can become necessary to suppress the function of the immune system with immunosuppressive drugs. On top of this, I read with horror that there was an increased risk of developing colon cancer in colitis patients and that surgical removal of the colon was a common procedure.

I was gutted. Until then, it had always been the others affected by severe illnesses. This horrible and seemingly desperate disease had suddenly slipped into our lives. I found that hard to accept. While doing my online research, I was careful that Luca was not looking over my shoulder and reading along with me. I was also glad that the nurse had mentioned nothing of this dark prognosis in Luca's presence. Luckily Luca, who otherwise would look up anything on the internet, did not get the idea to do his own research. I was depressed and highly concerned. However, I tried not to let it show.

For Luca, it was no question at all that he would soon be healthy again, and I did not want to destroy this firm belief. When Alex and I were lying in bed together late, I told him what I had found out about Luca's disease. I had the feeling that Alex tried to avoid allowing the information to get too close to him and that he somehow blocked it off. I felt infinitely sad. I simply could not accept that my child was supposed to be that ill all of a sudden. I cried myself into a restless sleep.

When I woke up the following day, it took a short moment until the thought of Luca's illness came back to my awareness. A feeling of desperation crushed me. Luca still could not take his medication. He made a new attempt. Until then, he did not have to swallow any pills. Drugs were almost taboo in our family, and we tried to avoid them as much as possible. Luca googled for tips on swallowing tablets that are far too big. He found out that other patients had the same problem with Asacolon as he did. In the meantime, I found out that the active substance mesalazine was also available in a granulated form. I asked myself why young patients weren't given the granules as the first option.

I inspected the information leaflet the nurse had given to me. It had been printed especially for Abbeytown Hospital, as it contained the nurse's name and contact details. At the bottom, I found the pharmaceutical company's name, which produces Asacolon in small print. Now I understood why this product was the first choice as the prescribed drug. There seemed to be a connection between this pharmaceutical company and the University Clinic.

In the brochure, I read that although the cause of IBD was unknown, there were indications that genetic factors and viral or bacterial infections could play a role in its causation. There would also be a link between an overreactive immune system and IBD. It was mentioned that psychological factors could trigger a flare-up. However, there was no indication they caused IBD.

I read about the several drug groups available as treatment options. Most of them were unknown to me. The list included steroids and 5-

ASA medications to which Luca's mesalazine drug belonged. Then it went on with immune modulators and biologics. Of course, the large number and severity of the side effects of these drugs caught my eye. They included allergic reactions, high blood pressure, stomach ulcers, damage of the lungs, and liver, kidney, and heart conditions.

Surgical procedures were mentioned as a further therapeutic intervention for ulcerative colitis and Crohn's disease. I was surprised that concerning ulcerative colitis, surgical removal of the colon and the creation of an artificial bowel outlet were talked about as if this was the most natural thing in the world. Patients were informed that after the operation, they could approach a specially trained nurse who would support them in managing their artificial bowel outlet. However, no negative impact on the patient's everyday life would usually have to be expected. It would be the doctor's decision whether the rectum was to be removed at the same time or if it remained with the patient for the moment and would be removed later.

I was horrified. I wondered how patients must feel when studying this "helpful information" on the day of their diagnosis. And how could it be pretended that this massive intervention would not impact the future lives of those affected? Having your colon removed and having to use a plastic bag that collects your faeces for the rest of your life is a significant impairment. Besides, a considerable part of the immune system is localised in the colon that is no longer present after the operation. On no account could we allow this to become Luca's future.

I refused to read this chapter of the leaflet to the end. What I had learnt sufficed to give me a terrible shock. I told Luca I would call the hospital the next day to get a new prescription for the granules. Nevertheless, he had the ambition to swallow the tablet. He probably thought he had no time to lose, as he wanted to recover as soon as possible. Finally, he overcame his aversion and managed to swallow the huge pill.

I spent almost the whole afternoon researching Luca's condition online. The thought of him having to take drugs with significant adverse effects for many years was hard to bear. At this time, an obvious question did not occur to me because I was too scared and almost paralysed: How could the nurse claim that Luca had to take the drugs for at least two years or longer? After all, she could not know how the illness would develop in Luca's case.

I didn't see why Luca should be "chronically" and, on top of that, "incurably" ill. Over a long time, he had supposedly made his symptoms up, and now, from one day to the next, he was allegedly chronically ill. The occurrence of his bloody diarrhoea was a relatively new thing.

How could it have become chronic already? I also had the impression that the term "chronic" was used synonymously with "incurable". That was not how I had understood the meaning of "chronic illness."

It also made little sense why the cause of Luca's symptoms should be entirely genetic. In everything I read, I encountered the same fatalistic attitude that was absolutely against my intuition. I doubted whether what we learnt about Luca's condition was the only way to see it. Again and again, a voice deep inside me said: "Luca will be healthy again." I was willing to do anything for him so he could get rid of this horrible disease.

3

Help for Self-Help

I googled "treating colitis naturally," and almost instantly, I came across the "Specific Carbohydrate Diet" and the book "Breaking the Vicious Cycle" by the biologist and nutritional scientist Elaine Gottschall. In retrospect, this precious find seems like providence to me. On the website for the book, I learnt more about its remarkable author, with whom I could easily identify. Just like me, Elaine Gottschall had been a mother who had refused to put up with the seemingly hopeless prognoses for her ill child and was not prepared to follow "expert" advice blindly.

At age four, her daughter Judy was diagnosed with severe ulcerative colitis. Despite continuous treatment with cortisone and sulfonamides, four years later, the surgical removal of a part of her gut seemed unavoidable. The Gottschalls were in absolute despair when they learnt about the New York-based paediatrician Dr Sidney Valentine Haas. He had successfully treated hundreds of children with celiac disease with the "Specific Carbohydrate Diet" (SCD) he developed. In 1951, he published the results of his therapy in his medical textbook "The Management of Celiac Disease." Dr Haas – aged 90 at the time – was the fifteenth physician consulted by the Gottschalls. He was the first one who wanted to know about their daughter's diet. Instead of the operation, he suggested the SCD as a therapy for Judy's colitis. From then on, Judy strictly followed this diet. Within a year, she was able to discontinue all her medication. As time progressed, Judy felt energetic and healthy again and was spared from the operation, which would have substantially impaired her life.

Whenever friends or people she knew were confronted with IBD, Elaine Gottschall felt the strong need to pass on her positive experiences with the SCD. However, she could not refer them to any doctors or scientists who supported treatment with this diet because, in the meantime, Dr Haas had died at the age of 94 in 1964. From then on, Elaine Gottschall devoted her life to helping patients with inflammatory bowel conditions. She was already 45 when she undertook the first steps to prepare for her biology and nutritional science studies. Elaine Gottschall wanted to achieve that medical professionals took the SCD seriously. From her own experience, she knew that the diet worked, but she wanted to study how it worked.

From 1975 to 1979, she studied at the Department of Cell Science at the University of Western Ontario. There she explored the effects of different sugars on the digestive tract. In 1979, she obtained her Master of Science degree. She worked at the University of Western Ontario Department of Anatomy the following year. She investigated the changes in the bowel wall of patients with inflammatory bowel conditions. In 1987 she self-published her first book, "Food and the Gut Reaction", of which she only sold 200 copies. She also attempted to inform the public about her findings in her many talks about the diet. After her guest appearance on a famous Canadian TV show, 23,000 copies of her book were sold within ten days, which she re-published under the title "Breaking the Vicious Cycle" in 1994. In the meantime, her book has been re-printed several times, translated into seven languages, and sold over a million times. Elaine Gottschall continued her public talks well into her old age. When she died in 2005, aged 84, she hoped that the results of her tireless work would not fall into oblivion.

The primary goals of the diet and how to reach them were easy to understand. The SCD eliminates all disaccharides, polysaccharides, and milk sugar (lactose) as patients cannot digest and absorb these sugars. Instead, they get into the colon, where they feed harmful bacteria. Because of this, they can multiply excessively. They produce metabolic products which are detrimental to the gut wall. In its attempt to protect itself against these harmful substances, the gut wall produces mucus in excess. That diminishes the gut's ability to absorb nutrients further, speeding up the increase of pathogenic microbes as they profit from the ample supply of nutrients. All of this creates a vicious cycle that the diet is supposed to break.

Although the SCD is very nutritious for the patient, it can starve out harmful microbes. Friendly bacteria, on the other hand, are being colonised in the gut by the intake of probiotics. These microorganisms support a healthy gut microbiome and the immune system associated with the gut. For this purpose, patients eat large amounts of homemade yoghurt, fermented for at least 24 hours.

Through the interplay of these interventions, the gut flora can gradually regain a healthy balance. Whereas this dietary approach can genuinely heal the gut, drugs only suppress the symptoms, and nothing changes regarding the root cause of the inflammation. Because of this, the patient remains ill. Could there have been a more convincing argument for introducing the SCD immediately?

I printed out a list of the foods that are allowed and those that are not permitted and studied them. The latter include grains and products made thereof, potatoes, rice, milk, certain types of cheese, sugar, and processed foods. I discussed the diet with Luca and asked if he wanted to try it. After all, it meant that he also had to give up all sweets. He did not hesitate for a second and said: "I will try anything if it helps me to become healthy again."

One reason was that he believed the diet would have a positive effect on his symptoms. But he also hoped the dietary changes would make him feel more energetic again, as he had felt exhausted long before the actual colitis symptoms. We were very optimistic; after all, we had nothing to lose. If the SCD had helped Gottschall's daughter and many other patients, why should it not help Luca? I ordered a copy of "Breaking the Vicious Cycle" immediately. The introduction diet was available on the website for the first days without the book and could be printed out. So it was possible to start right away.

It felt empowering that we didn't just have to put up with Luca's illness any longer. Now we could play an active role in regaining his health. The book gave us a nutrition guideline we could follow. On other websites, I found nutrition tips for colitis patients contradicting the SCD. These websites allowed potatoes and rice, for instance. However, I understood that the SCD excluded these foods because their polysaccharides were counter-productive to the abovementioned goals.

The SCD gave us new hope. I read that 75 per cent of the patients who followed it improved their condition. It sounded very promising. However, I also accepted that it was probably better for Luca to take his drugs until he had achieved a more prolonged remission. Taking the medication and following the diet were not mutually exclusive after all. At this point, I was not ready to take over the responsibility of simply discontinuing the medication. In her book, Gottschall advices doing this only in consultation with a physician.

In the evening, I helped Luca with the Salofalk enema. I was not pleased with the listed side effects, but I decided to accept them for the moment. I hoped they would not occur in Luca's case. I had not realised then that there are no real "side" effects. "Side effects" are mostly not desired but are part of a drug's effects, just like the ones you want to achieve. I did not mention them to Luca, as I did not want to burden him. He had been worried about his health for too long already.

At the beginning of his puberty, he kept complaining about pains in the chest area. These occurred for the first time after he had suffered from a circulatory collapse in connection with the Mendel-Mantoux tuberculin test. This tuberculosis skin test was part of a vaccination campaign against tuberculosis that the Irish Health Service HSE had carried out through Irish schools. When Luca left the clinic after the test, for which tuberculin was injected intradermally in the lower part of the arm, he started feeling dizzy and fainted. Luca was twelve years old then and was afraid he would die. This event shocked him immensely. Luca was not the only child who suffered adverse effects. The clinic was prepared for this as there was a room where the respective children could lie down and rest. Yet nobody had informed the parents beforehand that this could happen.

I met with the responsible doctor a few days after Luca's experience. I wanted to talk to her about the necessity of a tuberculosis vaccine because I did not see a substantiated reason for it. I mentioned to her that Luca had fainted after the tuberculin test. She explained that men, in particular, could be prone to fainting, for instance, when their blood is taken. She said that Luca could be such a "fainter" and that it would be better if he lay down on such an occasion in the future.

However, Luca had never fainted before or after the tuberculin test. Only a few years later, I learnt that the tuberculin test could contain phenol, a highly poisonous and mutagen chemical substance. Fainting (syncope) is a known adverse reaction of the cardiovascular system to the tuberculin test. Maybe there was no connection between Luca's chest pain and the tuberculin test, but it started after this traumatic event, and Luca interpreted it as heart pain. Dr Morrin could not observe any abnormalities during an electrocardiogram, so he believed Luca's symptoms were growing pains.

Years later, Luca told me that during this time, he had often been lying in his bed with chest pains at night. He had been crying because he was afraid not to wake up again the following day. I asked him why he had never told us about it. Luca answered that no one had believed him anyway. It was a very stressful time for him, and he worried about his heart for many years. This worry developed into a "heart phobia".

Regarding his health, the tuberculin test marked the beginning of a downward spiral for Luca. I don't know whether the ingredients were directly responsible for it, whether the traumatic experience of fainting had triggered it, or whether both factors worked together. However, Luca told me that his syncope and experience afterwards had taken the illusion of invulnerability away from him. Deep faith in our invulnerability is essential for our health, especially at a young age.

Maybe Luca's "heart phobia" also explains why Dr Morrin had not taken the symptoms leading up to Luca's colitis more seriously. He probably labelled him as a "hypochondriac". Maybe he also thought that the symptoms described by Luca were just an excuse to avoid school. However, daily diarrhoea, burning abdominal pain, frequent heartburn, and permanently congested nasal cavities are alarm signals a doctor must pursue. They point to dysbiosis – a dysfunctional gut microbiome – and this pathology or deviation of normal physiology precedes ulcerative colitis. Unfortunately, our GP failed concerning Luca's treatment. He could have spared Luca and us from a lot of trouble with more competence and foresight. I am convinced about that today.

Because of Luca's history, I was afraid he could "make up" adverse effects, so I did not mention them to him. However, I wanted to keep an eye on him concerning any occurring side effects. On the next day, I succeeded in reaching the nurse by phone. I informed her that Luca had difficulty swallowing the tablets and asked if he could take the granules instead. She offered to send me a new prescription by post.

I told her that Luca would start with the introduction of the SCD and explained to her the goals of this diet. I asked her if she could support us with implementing the diet in any way. The nurse said she had never heard about a "Specific Carbohydrate Diet". She said that patients must find out by themselves which foods they can tolerate. In principle, however, nutrition would not play a role in the genesis of the disease. It would be an absolute must for Luca to take his medication for at least two years, if not for the rest of his life, she added.

Furthermore, because of an increased risk of developing colon cancer, getting into remission with the help of medication would be essential. I had read all of this several times before. I thanked her for sending me the new prescription and said goodbye.

After I had put down the receiver, I reflected on our conversation again. The hospital in Abbeytown was an Irish University Clinic. The nurse was Dr Cody's right hand and the patient's first contact point. How could she have never heard about a diet which had helped thousands of patients worldwide with Crohn's disease or ulcerative colitis? Again and again, I heard the same thing from medical professionals: They claimed that a patient's diet had nothing to do with IBD. From the very beginning, this contradicted my intuition and common sense. Was it possible that there was a system behind all of this? At any rate, it did not serve the patients' welfare but the pharmaceutical companies' financial interests.

"There's no profit in proving that diet can be used to help the millions of IBDers who take daily medication or need surgery and a steady supply of ostomy bags. Therefore, doctors present most patients with limited options (1)," is how SCD-activist, colitis-patient, and author Raman Prasad summed up the situation in his book, "Colitis & Me".

I was determined to try the diet with Luca and discontinue his medications step by step as soon as he would be better. After all, he was only sixteen. Being on drugs for the rest of his life was not a good prospect for him. Even only the thought of it was a horror to me. It also did not align with Luca's self-image. He did not want to become a "medication junky". It simply did not make sense that a child, who had had a healthy lifestyle most of his life, should suddenly be so ill that there was no hope for a cure.

I could see that Luca's diet had not been very versatile lately. I also knew that his meals consisted of exactly those foods eliminated from his diet now, namely grains in the form of bread, pasta, oat crackers and cereals, and plenty of sugar. I had mentioned my suspicion to Dr Morrin several times that there had to be a connection between all those grains and Luca's symptoms. However, he had tried to put me at ease by saying that Luca's test for celiac disease was negative, meaning he could not have any problems with grains. However, some colitis patients respond well to eliminating gluten from their diet and can even be cured, although antibodies indicating celiac disease could not be found in their blood.

We gradually introduced the SCD, and when the book landed in our letter box only a few days later, we started properly. I also started keeping a special diary in which I noted what Luca had consumed, whether he had suffered from flatulence, how many bowel movements he had, what their consistency was like, and how he felt in general. That allowed me to always trace back possible triggers for his body's reactions, even though they dated back a few days. Gottschall explicitly points out that the SCD has to be strictly followed if you want to succeed. Usually, there would be a change in bowel movements after a few days on this diet. However, it would take three to four weeks until an improvement in the condition could be seen. If this were not the case, it would be possible that the patient was not responsive to the SCD.

It was the first time that I had prepared homemade yoghurt. As I didn't have a yoghurt maker yet, I fermented the yoghurt in the oven overnight with the oven light switched on and a hot water bottle as an additional heat source. The yoghurt smelled delicious and somehow comforting. Moreover, it simply tasted wonderful. "SCD yoghurt" has to be fermented for at least 24 hours. The lactic acid bacteria, which are added to the milk, digest the milk sugar (lactose) present in the milk and multiply. When the yoghurt is ready, it no longer contains any lactose. Lactose is indigestible for certain people, as they lack the necessary digestive enzymes. Instead of lactose, this homemade yoghurt contains billions of gut-friendly probiotic microorganisms, which is not the case with commercial products. I thought about the fact that Luca never really liked drinking milk. Sometimes it even made him feel sick. Yoghurt, on the other hand, he always wanted to eat. However, commercial yoghurt does not necessarily contain any live bacteria; in most cases, it is also sweetened.

I also made broth from chicken or beef bones and vegetables and prepared soup for Luca. The animal bones and cartilage contain collagen with anti-inflammatory and immunomodulating properties and can heal a leaky gut. For this reason, I also made "SCD jelly", which Luca loved to eat with SCD yoghurt. It consisted of unsweetened natural apple juice and beef gelatine powder.

Since the mad cow disease, gelatine and beef bones were taboo in our household. Therefore, I had to force myself to use gelatine. I had never expected that it contained substances with therapeutic effects. Was it possible to heal with a goal-oriented utilisation of foods? I remember that homemade broth was served as a starter in my grandmother's household before every dinner. She neither knew what collagen was nor that it supports a healthy gut. Nonetheless, in her generation, it was common knowledge that eating bone broth before dinner was good for you.

4

Food as Medicine

"Let your food be your medicine, and your medicine be your food."
(Hippocrates, 460–370 BC)

Two days after Luca's dietary changes, his energy levels were significantly higher. Only six days after the colonoscopy, no more visible blood was in his stool. He only had two bowel movements per day and no longer had to run to the toilet. The following day, he only went to the bathroom once, and his stool had a firmer consistency. Luca was feeling very well. He liked his new diet, which gave him a feeling of satiety that he hadn't experienced in a long time.

I had spent almost all day preparing his food and washing pots and pans. The diet preparation turned out to be very time-consuming and labour-intensive, as I had to prepare everything from scratch. Although I had never really used ready-made meals, bread and pasta are also convenience foods that save us plenty of time in the kitchen.

If we took the implementation of the SCD seriously, it would demand a lot of work input from my side and a lot of discipline from Luca's. However, if the reward was that we could win back his health, I was ready for anything. I also asked myself if I could feed Luca without bread and the usual pasta, rice, or potatoes on the side. Over time, however, it turned out that high-quality fats are filling and satisfying.

I had arranged another appointment with Dr Morrin to discuss Luca's diagnosis and blood values. I took the opportunity to inform him about our dietary approach and told him that Luca was feeling quite well again. Dr Morrin was unfamiliar with the SCD and pointed out that there were *so many* diets on the internet. I felt I was not taken seriously and answered that this was not just *any* diet. I explained that the SCD had been proven effective since the first half of the last century and that it was clinically tried and tested. I added that it was supposed to have a success rate of 75 per cent.

At least Dr Morrin was prepared to google the book title "Breaking the Vicious Cycle" immediately. I don't know if he only did it out of politeness or if he looked into the diet again later. I explained to him that playing an active role and taking the proper steps to support Luca's healing process meant a lot to me. I also told him I was apprehensive about the drugs' adverse effects. Once again, he tried to reassure me. He said he had a sister with colitis in Australia who had achieved great results with the drugs. It made me wonder. If he had a sister with colitis, how could he not have known there was blood in the stool of colitis patients?

I asked myself if this sister existed at all and which other diseases she might have apart from colitis. Dr Morrin was probably well-meaning in trying to put my mind at ease, but he did not exactly inspire my confidence in him. He explained to me that from now on, Luca had to come for blood tests regularly. It would be necessary to check if he had any vitamin or mineral deficiencies. Besides, it would be required to exclude that he was anaemic and losing occult blood, which means that it is not visible to us. Moreover, it would have to be ensured that the medication did not damage Luca's liver or kidneys.

In her book, Elaine Gottschall recommended implementing the diet in cooperation with the attending physician. We would have wished for this, but obviously, we could not expect any support from our doctors. Luca and I had to see this through on our own. In the meantime, I have learnt that doctors without a holistic approach simply haven't a clue about nutrition. Their curriculum is not designed to gain a thorough understanding of this domain in Germany, Ireland, or the USA. However, it hasn't always been that way. With the increasing use of drugs, an adequate diet as a therapeutic approach has been pushed increasingly into the background.

Despite our immediate success with the SCD, I asked myself if it was the most suitable diet for Luca. Therefore, I made an appointment with an alternative practitioner I knew. Moni is also from Germany and has been living in Ireland for decades. I told her about Luca's illness, the SCD, and our previous experiences. Only then I realised how stressed and mentally strained I was. I could not suppress my tears and an outburst of emotion. "Why did it have to be Luca who got this dreadful disease?"

Moni took me in her arms. I told her that it wasn't doing me any good to research mainstream health websites representing orthodox medicine's point of view. It would frighten me a lot. I told her that I was horrified that Luca might get his colon removed sometime in the future and that he would have to live with a plastic bag for his stool for the rest of his life.

"This won't happen. Just don't read these websites. The pharmaceutical industry, with its brainwashing and attempts at intimidation, is behind this. You will get a grip on Luca's illness. He is still so young. Every cell of his body is constantly being renewed; within seven years, all of the cells have been renewed. He will learn what is good for him and what isn't." She wasn't familiar with the SCD, but from what I had told her about it, it made a lot of sense to her. "You are on the right track. However, you also have to look after your own health! Luca shall help you in the kitchen." I was very grateful for Moni's encouragement and the reassurance she gave me.

We constantly integrated new permitted foods and meals into Luca's diet. In the beginning, for instance, he ate scrambled eggs with cooked and mashed apples or pears, minced meat with puréed butternut pumpkin, chicken breast or cod with carrots, and of course, chicken soup. I used turmeric as often as possible as a spice for its anti-inflammatory effects. Between meals, Luca drank ginger tea, which has anti-inflammatory properties also, and fennel or peppermint tea. On the eleventh day after his diagnosis, Luca had no bowel movements at all, and from then on, his stools were normal again. Also, the horrible smelling "slurry farts", which announced new flare-ups and were present during an active disease phase, had disappeared entirely.

Luca was in good form. He waited another while until he started his football training again but decided to edit a new football video from footage he already had. Luca was emotionally balanced and had the patience to view his video material for hours and create an editing plan. He taught himself how to use the professional editing programme I had on my laptop without any difficulties. I thought it was great how easy he found it. Things were also going well with the diet. In the meantime, I bought a yoghurt maker, which allowed me to prepare two litres of yoghurt in one go.

Step by step, we extended the diet by

introducing courgettes, honeydew melons, and cheddar. On the tenth day of the diet, I made pork chops with carrots, butternut pumpkin, and apple pieces on a baking tray in the oven. We were all eating from it and liked it. On the following day, Luca had several bowel movements. I was worried if it might have been a bit early for pork chops yet and if they might be too hard to digest for him at this point. As he was feeling very well otherwise and as he had started to train football again, this might have stimulated his gut activity.

Because Luca was practising sports again, we sought a convenient snack that provided energy between his meals. Luca tried it with cheddar and cashew nuts. Of course, bananas were always a good snack too. Luca was especially fond of the pancakes I treated him to every morning for breakfast. The batter consisted of coconut flour and mashed bananas. I baked them with ghee (clarified butter) or organic virgin coconut oil. He ate them with cooked, puréed pears, SCD yoghurt, and honey. I also made kebabs with tiny meatballs, cheese, and cherry tomatoes for him. He always welcomed chicken or turkey breast as well. A variation of this was a stir fry in combination with courgettes, carrots, and peppers. A casserole made from cubed steak, carrots, and pumpkin, cooked very slowly, also went down well with him.

When Luca had been on the SCD for two and a half weeks, I finally wanted to bake something for him. It would take some pressure from me if Luca could eat a slice of almond flour bread sometimes. For its preparation, I bought whole almonds, which I blanched, peeled, and dried before I ground them into almond flour. Elaine Gottschall recommended this in her book, at least at the start of the diet, to avoid industrially ground and processed almonds.

Luca was a model patient who strictly followed his diet and never forgot to take his medication. I could be one hundred per cent sure that he would never eat anything which was not permitted, but apparently, he didn't find it hard. The honey he ate with his pancakes in the mornings satisfied his desire for something sweet. Honey also has therapeutic effects because it is anti-inflammatory. Luca didn't regret a single time that he wasn't allowed to eat sweets any longer. He told me that he had never really liked bread and pasta and that cake often had given him heartburn or acid reflux. All those sweets had caused him a bad conscience because he feared they could harm his health. He knew that the foods he had been eating were not aligned with his athletic ambitions. He said he was glad that he was following a different diet now. It would have been a good idea to listen to what his body or subconscious mind had told him all along much earlier!

Luca just loved the food I made for him. He also rediscovered the delicious flavours of all the different vegetables. Everything tasted much more intensive for him now. Sugar and industrially processed foods manipulate our natural sense of taste and don't let us notice any longer what our body really needs. As an infant, Luca liked almost every kind of vegetable. The large amounts of sweet things that children consume spoil their appetite for vegetables, and all of a sudden, they don't like them anymore.

When preparing the diet, it is essential not to over-boil the vegetables. Firstly, they taste better when they are still a bit crunchy; secondly, you don't lose as many of their precious vitamins. Besides, you preserve the different colours of the vegetables, which is a prerequisite for presenting a meal in a visually attractive manner. The more colours you have on your plate, the healthier your meal is. Eat the rainbow! A varied diet also supports the diversity of our intestinal microbiome. And this has a positive effect on our gut health, our immune system, our psyche, and our general well-being.

5

Riding High

December 2016

One month had passed since Luca had started implementing the SCD. He noticed that he had not felt as good, balanced, and energetic for ages. The acid reflux symptoms, which Luca had suffered from for a long time, had disappeared. He also did not constantly feel hungry; when he was hungry, he did not have a burning sensation in the gut region, followed by diarrhoea. Luca's stool was completely normal again and wasn't a conversation topic anymore. Before the diet, Luca had also suffered from night blindness which can be a sign of vitamin A deficiency. Now he could see silhouettes in the darkness again, which is normal. His nasal sinuses were no longer blocked, and when he spoke, it did not sound like he was holding his nose.

We had a follow-up appointment at the University hospital with Dr Cody. He wanted to discuss the result of the colonoscopy with us. He said that Luca's entire colon had been inflamed but not severely. The tissue samples he had taken had not shown any abnormalities. Dr Cody asked how Luca was feeling now. We told him he was very well and that we were convinced this was also due to his diet. Dr Cody was unfamiliar with the SCD but was open and recommended that we continue with it.

He said Luca could discontinue the Salofalk enemas he had applied for four weeks. However, Luca should continue to take the granules. Dr Cody added that this medication was safe and well tolerated as it wasn't a steroid and because its function was limited to the intestines. I doubted it was possible to determine the effect of a drug on a specific location in the body. If this medicine only impacted the intestines, why was it necessary to have regular blood tests to check that they didn't damage the liver or the kidneys? Contradictions like this did not exactly contribute to a trusting relationship between Luca's consultant and us. We were relieved that Luca was already able to reduce his drugs. He was glad to get rid of the rectal medication, which he had named "ass trumpet" because he had found its application unpleasant and awkward.

Driving through busy Abbeytown on our way back, the Christmas decorations and light chains reminded us of Christmas being just around the corner. There were only ten days left until Christmas Eve. There had never been an Advent season without Christmas goodies in our family before. Out of consideration for Luca, Alex and I abstained from German "lebkuchen", "stollen", "spekulatius", and other sweet pastries and substituted these traditional Christmas treats with a handful of nuts or dried fruits. We wanted to back

Luca through our solidarity. Alex found it a lot more challenging to do without than myself.

During the introduction phase of the diet, I went food shopping in Lidl and looked at all the shelves filled with Christmas treats when I caught myself feeling pity for Luca. All of this, he was not allowed to eat anymore. However, when I started thinking critically about all this unhealthy junk, my feeling of pity disappeared quickly. In addition to vast amounts of sugar, it contains unhealthy fats, emulsifiers, artificial colourings, and preservatives. However, I regretted not having any Christmas cookies for the festive season. I had always made biscuits, which were part of our family's Christmas tradition.

I searched for "SCD-biscuits" on the internet and came across the fantastic, inspiring website of the American Raman Prasad. (See the list of websites at the end of this book.) At the age of 17, Prasad was diagnosed with ulcerative colitis. He described his long history of suffering and his final healing journey with the SCD in his autobiographical report "Colitis & Me". Elaine Gottschall wrote the foreword to this book. Both shared a deep friendship, and Prasad is one of the SCD devotees who dedicated themselves to promoting this diet to carry the message further. He is also the author of SCD cooking books and generously makes many recipes available on his website. Here I found recipes for focaccia and almond biscuits. I was thrilled. I would bake these for all of us for Christmas!

Gradually our life returned to normality. There was hardly any time left for my interests or work as a freelance translator. I was upset about it, but the main thing was that Luca was feeling well again. I was convinced that one day his colitis would no longer be an issue for us. Before Christmas, Luca wanted to go to his hairdresser in Abbeytown. In the previous months, his outer appearance had become relatively unimportant to him, but now he felt like getting a good haircut. Besides, his Hungarian barber, who had been cutting his hair for years, was his only remaining friend. All his former school friends had withdrawn from Luca.

Christmas was nearing. This year, we didn't have as much money as usual, but this shouldn't stop us from celebrating a wonderful Christmas together. Alex and I did more or less without any presents. I only wanted Kate Bush's new live album, which I had longingly awaited for quite some time. Luca ordered the gifts he wanted online: a high-quality match ball, new freestyle football shoes, and a few items of stylish training gear.

My aim was that Christmas would be as it had always been. I didn't want Luca to feel that things were any different just because of his illness. We saved the money for a Christmas tree by Alex felling one of the many large pine trees in our small wood. He sawed the top part off, and the resulting Christmas tree was massive, a real nature bloke about three metres high with a corresponding diameter and ivy trailing up its trunk. Luca and I decorated it together. The decorations reminded us of all the happy and harmonious Christmases we had celebrated together.

We waited with the presents until Christmas Day according to the Irish tradition. We spent the day in a relaxed way and didn't open our presents until after lunch. Like every year, we had salmon with brown bread, which Alex and I enjoyed with a glass of Guinness. For Luca, I had baked the focaccia, which tasted absolutely delicious with the salmon.

That year the presents under the Christmas tree had not been as abundant as in the previous years when I still had been able to work. However, Luca was feeling very well again, and this was more important than anything else. We also didn't have to do without our traditional Christmas dinner, which Luca had always loved. We had turkey and oven-roasted ham with honey glazing and cloves. (We cheated a little here because the SCD does not permit cured meats.) With this, we had various types of vegetables on the side and cranberry sauce which I had made myself this year. The only food that Luca was not allowed to eat was potatoes. Instead of the usual Irish Christmas pudding, I made energy balls from dried fruits and almonds.

Especially the Medjool dates, which I had bought instead of chocolate, tasted heavenly.

Luca also ate fresh fruits again, which inspired me to prepare a fruit salad. Despite the diet, Luca didn't feel like missing out on anything. We had a relaxed and merry Christmas together. Filled with optimism, I noted in my colitis diary: *The colitis, which has caused us so much distress and worries, will no longer be an issue soon.*

Luca had put on a few kilograms. He looked healthy and well, and his face was fuller again. He was back to training every day, which benefited his overall well-being. It was essential for him to know that the colitis would not be in his way of fulfilling his dream of becoming a professional footballer. We considered it a necessity that he consumed more calories. Therefore we decided to integrate permitted pulses like lentils and beans into his diet.

"It is not happy people who are grateful. It is grateful people who are happy."
(Francis Bacon, 1561–1626)

Luca wished to have pizza as dinner for New Year's Eve. I discovered a recipe for pizza in "Breaking the Vicious Cycle" and prepared it. Luca was delighted by the crunchy pizza base I made from almond flour. This pizza not only tastes fantastic but is also very nutritious. We decided to let the old year sound out with the new Kate Bush CD, which we listened to for the first time with great enthusiasm. Afterwards, we watched our favourite music show, "Later with Jools Holland". We were all glad to say bye-bye to the old year and welcome the new one. As Luca's recovery progressed so well and we were on the way up again, we had high hopes that the New Year would be better than the previous one.

6

Crushed

On New Year's Day, I tried out a kind of Curry. The ingredients were chicken breast, broccoli, lentils, tomatoes, coconut milk from the tin, freshly ground ginger and fresh coriander. I soaked the lentils overnight as recommended by the SCD. All of us enjoyed this dish very much. It was also practical because we could all eat it. It spared me from cooking two different meals.

However, the following morning, I noticed that somehow the food had disagreed with me. I hoped that Luca would not feel the same. Alex and I decided to drive to the town of Ogham for some shopping. I was happy about this rare occasion to get out and see something other than pots and pans. The short overland journey felt very liberating. I realised I had to create a little more freedom for myself again.

When we came home in the evening, Luca was sitting in front of the television with a stern face. He told me that his belly was feeling kind of funny. I reassured him and said I had not felt great in the morning either. I added that nobody was feeling the same every day. After all, the human body was not a machine but a living organism. In retrospect, I ask myself why I again offered the same food to Luca that evening. Heated up and cooked for a little longer, it tasted much better. I assumed the lentils had not been properly done on the previous day. At the end of the week, we had another pizza with tinned tomatoes.

Shortly after, Luca had another mild flare-up with several diarrhoea-like stools over the day, however, without any blood. We were very alarmed. Luca completely lost his usual rhythm. The days were extremely short – there was daylight for seven hours only – and Luca slept until 2 pm. However, he didn't go to bed until after midnight and was also hungry again at night-time. For me, this meant working in the kitchen until midnight often. It was highly demanding, and I perceived it as unfair that claiming back Luca's health was so hard. But then I said to myself that self-pity would not help much and that I should be grateful to be able to support Luca. Luca's health was my priority, even if it meant that I missed out.

We were already in the second week of January. I hoped that Luca would soon be better again. I decided to take down the remaining Christmas decorations and tidy up a little to distract myself. Then the bloody diarrhoea returned. Luca said: "It's like when a hated person you thought you'd never have to see again in your life suddenly shows up on your doorstep." It was a terrible falloff for us. With the help of the diet, things had gone steeply uphill for weeks, and we had felt that it would continue like this forever. We had been on a real high. Now we embraced one another, crying. On top of the annual anticlimax after Christmas and the dark season, we had to deal with Luca's flare-up.

Luca remembered that somewhere in his room, there had to be a leftover Salofalk enema. He insisted on applying it and on using this medication again. Luca spent the night in the living room in an armchair in front of the fire. In this position, he found it easier to bear his abdominal pain. He hardly slept, and I also spent a restless night where my thoughts went round and round in circles non-stop. I felt tremendously sorry for Luca. Up to then, everything had worked out so well. Why were we punished like this? Why had the symptoms returned? Could it be that I had not been careful enough with the diet?

In my head, I went through everything again, which might have caused Luca any problems. Luca had not eaten anything that was not permitted, but it may have been too early for some of the ingredients, for instance, the cashews. And the lentils with which we should have waited until after being on the SCD for three months. I also should have avoided the tinned tomatoes, as they can contain hidden sugars. Tinned coconut milk was not a good idea either, as it contains xanthan gum, which I only found out afterwards. This thickening- and stabilising agent can cause adverse reactions in the gut, and patients with inflammatory bowel disease should avoid it. Of course, this made me wonder why this substance was contained in Luca's rectal medication then.

The next day, I felt weak and exhausted and constantly cried. I was terribly frustrated. The diagnosis, two months earlier, had by far not thrown me off balance as much. During the past few weeks, I had been convinced that Luca would get healthy again with the help of the diet. How pleased we had been with our success. Now I felt like someone had pulled the rug out from under me.

Before this new flare-up and while Luca had been in better form, I had discontinued my internet research. I did not want to be preoccupied with his illness all the time. I was happy that a kind of normality had returned to our lives. Now the time started again, during which I spent every spare minute in front of my laptop, obsessed with my research. I found out that there are four to six new ulcerative colitis patients per 100,000 inhabitants in Germany every year. For Crohn's disease, the annual incidence rate is between six and seven individuals per 100,000 inhabitants. *(1)*

Seemingly, the risk of getting ulcerative colitis is reduced by 70 per cent if an individual has been breastfed and has grown up with pets. Both factors applied to Luca. I nurtured him until he was two years old. We owned a dog, a cat, and chickens;

we even had donkeys for some time.

So I kept asking myself: "Why Luca?" I imagined an alpine area of 100,000 square meters with four to six glacial crevasses. Why did my child have to fall into such a crevasse, although I had always attempted to do everything "right"? It was like an endless tape that I kept playing in my head repeatedly. My fair-world belief had been badly shaken up, and I was well on my way to becoming embittered. But I couldn't allow Luca's illness to break me. He needed me so much.

During the following days, Luca and I suffered very bad spells of feeling depressed. Whoever was momentarily in better shape tried to encourage the other. Again and again, we kept telling each other how much we loved one another. When Luca noticed I was in despair, he consoled me with the words: "We are doing everything right. Everything will be fine again." – "Yes, everything will be good," I reassured him. From now on, this became our mantra. However, Luca was very sad and frustrated. He had firmly believed that with the help of the diet and his medications, he would soon be perfectly healthy again. I deliberately had never told him that his illness was supposed to be "chronic" and "incurable".

7

Doubt and Hope

About conventional Western medicine, it has often been stated that you cannot beat it in the field of emergency care. However, the picture is entirely different when it comes to addressing chronic disease. Besides medication, our doctors had nothing to offer Luca so far to support his healing journey. If I wanted him to be able to reverse his illness, I had to educate myself and get as independent from our doctors as possible. My most pressing question was whether Luca could become healthy again.

I often did night shifts trying to find answers on the internet. Afterwards, my head was spinning with all the information, and despite feeling completely exhausted, I could not find restful sleep.

I discovered that Cork University College in the South-East of Ireland has a renowned microbiome institute. I decided to write an email to one of its professors. His field of research was how the microbiome affects the psyche. I informed him that Luca was suffering from colitis and asked him for his opinion.

I explained to him that I saw Luca's unfavourable diet and extensive stress as triggers for his condition. I described Luca's diet before the onset of the colitis symptoms and told him about my suspicion that it had damaged his gut microbiome, resulting in a leaky gut. I also informed him that Luca had been suffering from an anxiety disorder for the past three years and that, momentarily, he was suffering from a contamination phobia. I explained that I guessed that Luca's fear of becoming contaminated raised the alert state of his immune system and that his "intestinal brain" mirrored this fear. I mentioned the SCD to him and told him about our success with it so far. I asked him if our experience with the diet was of any interest to the scientific research at the institute. I explained that I would be happy to make our experience available and to keep him up to date with our progress. In return, I was hoping to receive competent support.

Maybe it was naïve even vaguely to expect an answer, but I did not care. I had nothing to lose. To my surprise, I already found the professor's reply in my mailbox the following morning. He fully supported my interpretation of the causes of Luca's colitis and advised therapy with probiotics. He wished us that Luca would have a complete recovery. I floated with happiness, and I was infinitely grateful for his feedback. I felt confirmed in my belief that we were on the right path and that Luca could become healthy again. During my further research on the internet, I discovered a newspaper article written by a colitis patient. After years of unsuccessful medical therapy, she had cured herself with the Specific Carbohydrate Diet. This article gave me a further uplift. I realised the importance of making a healing success like this public to counter the biased and narrow-minded view of conventional medicine and the information given by the pharmaceutical industry.

Luca's present flare-up had already been going on for six days, and I let him sleep until the late afternoon. As is well known, rest is the best medicine. But I was hoping that Luca would not be standing beside my bed in the middle of the night again, telling me he was hungry. The recurrence of the symptoms had taken a lot out of him. On some days, he slept 16 hours in one go. I had not yet realised that his medication could also have contributed to his extreme tiredness. Fatigue is only one of many side effects of mesalazine (5-aminosalicylic acid).

However, Luca's health started improving again, and he felt a little better day by day. He only had one daily bowel movement, and we could reduce the alert level. I showed Luca how to prepare his pancakes. From now on, he made his own breakfast. I researched alternative remedies and dietary supplements for colitis therapy, of which there is quite a number. Besides curcumin, I learned about bromelain and Boswellia extract, which constitute promising natural remedies. I would have liked to use alternative natural therapeutic products but did not know which ones to choose. I was also uncertain if they were compatible with Luca's drugs.

However, all in all, my research confirmed my feeling that we were on the right track with the SCD. We had good reason to be optimistic. Nevertheless, I was emotionally and mentally completely burnt out. I hated this disease, no matter what had caused it. It ruined our lives. I had turned into an outright crybaby and had to weep constantly.

One morning I woke up with a migraine. When I looked in the mirror, I discovered a bruise under one of my eyes which looked like a black eye. I probably had cried too much, and a small blood vessel had burst. The face that looked back at me from the mirror seemed like it had turned to stone. This wasn't me, was it? For heaven's sake! It couldn't go on like this. Despite all my efforts, there was no change in my state of mind on this day either. I suffered from mood swings, and although I did not want to cry as much any more, the tears just kept running for no direct reason. "Mama, I love you!" Luca often said to me. "I love you too, Luca," I replied and tried to smile at him. Then he wanted to cheer me up: "I am all right again. We are doing everything right."

Maybe at this point, it was harder for me to cope with his relapse than for Luca. In my imagination, the path back to health probably had seemed too easy, and I had overlooked that the regeneration of Luca's gut would take a very long time. I knew it did not contribute to Luca's healing if he constantly saw me with a worried face or crying. Therefore I told myself that I had to focus on all the positive things and that I had to believe very strongly in the diet's success.

Luca's appetite had returned, which meant I had to spend more time with the practical side of his diet again. When I was feeling stressed, I tried to breathe deep into my belly, hold my breath for a while, and breathe out through my mouth again. That helped me to reduce my stress levels, at least for some time. I also tried encouraging Luca to do this 4–7–8 breathing exercise, as I was sure it would benefit him.

On the following day, Luca also slept very long. In the evening, he discovered a slight trace of blood in his stool and was very low-spirited. Luca feared everything would start all over again. He was terribly nervous and anxious, and I felt extremely sorry for him. Constantly these worries and this fear. He was still a child, after all. Why did he have to suffer so much? Why could he not have an easy-going life like other young people?

But maybe he was not like "the others" and did not want to be like them anymore. Being the only German among Irish children, he had never felt like being part of them. He had tried to compensate for his insecurity by over-adapted behaviour, always wanting to do it right for everybody else. In friendships, he had always felt like the fifth wheel on the wagon under which he had suffered for years. Luca was two and a half years old when Alex and I decided to fulfil our big dream: moving to Ireland. We had wished a happy childhood for Luca, but we had bestowed lonesome childhood years upon him.

For Luca, Germany had always remained his true homeland. When he was small, he always said before falling asleep: "I want to go home." Puzzled, I replied: "But you are at home." Only now do I realise that the roots Alex and I had given him within our family had not been sufficient to ground him.

If you compare the human body with a tree, the intestine with its villi corresponds to the root system. With its roots, a plant absorbs nutrients from the ground, and soil bacteria help it to make these nutrients usable. A further parallel to the human gut is that the microorganisms in the soil train the plant's immune system. For the human immune system, the gut bacteria take over this role. In Ayurvedic medicine, the colon and the immune system are associated with the root chakra. Chakras are the psycho-spiritual energy centres in the human body. In the root chakra at the base of the spine, our basic trust is supposed to be located, but in Luca's case, there was a lot of fear.

I became increasingly aware that Luca's symptoms mirrored his inner condition and that somatic (bodily), mental, emotional and social factors are deeply intertwined and constantly interact. The extent to which these factors are involved in an individual's disease can vary significantly from one person to another.

Luca's symptoms seemed to me like a self-fulfilling prophecy. Before the first occurrence of his bloody diarrhoea, he had been convinced for a long time that his body was being contaminated. He was sure that he had contaminated our home with his school utensils. He made the chemicals from his chemistry class responsible for this contamination.

As the tables in the science room were always wet and sticky, he believed that this mess originated from spilt chemicals. To make matters even worse, one of his classmates had deliberately poured a beaker with stale chemicals over Luca's backpack and shoes. He feared that he had taken small traces of the "poison" back to our home and that they were spread all over the place. As a result, he would also contaminate himself at home.

For this reason, he no longer ate anything with his hands but only with cutlery that he had rinsed under running water beforehand. He feared that he was doing irreparable damage to his body by the constant accumulation of toxins. This damage might only get apparent years later and would then be irreversible.

I shouldn't have told Alex and Luca about the leaky gut syndrome. By doing this, I had fuelled

Luca's anxiety even more. Now he believed the "school poison" would pass through his leaky gut into his bloodstream. Despite our endless discussions, I couldn't talk him out of his convictions. He not only had to deal with his gut symptoms but also with his deep-rooted fear, which put him under permanent stress. That, again, affected what was going on in his gut. Luca constantly observed me while I was working in the kitchen. He controlled that I was doing everything "right" and that I did not touch his food with "contaminated" hands. Sometimes, I didn't know what was worse, his colitis or his contamination phobia, but both aspects belonged together and were closely interlinked.

Since his recent flare-up, twelve days had passed. Luca had not left the house this whole time and still needed a lot of sleep. However, when he was awake, he felt good and was always ready for a joke. There were still a few tiny red dots in his stool, which was firmer again. I reassured Luca that this meant that the inflammation was slowly coming to an end. Luca's body was still very weak from the last attack. Otherwise, he would have taken a ball in his hands or better on his feet long ago. His footballs had been abandoned somewhere in a corner which was not typical for Luca at all.

On the following days, he also slept almost until dusk. Although I had arranged an appointment with our GP in the morning, I knew that Luca would not be able to get up early. It didn't matter; I would go alone and bombard Dr Morrin with questions.

In the meantime, I had become quite annoyed with him. In my opinion, he had been sleeping for the past few years. As a doctor, he should have investigated why Luca had been complaining about having no energy for so long. And this, although he had been eating enough. He had never asked a single question about Luca's diet.

I assumed that by now, I knew more about nutrition than our doctor. And I was expanding my knowledge about it continuously. While researching online, I discovered Dr Campbell-McBride's GAPS diet and her article "Gut and Psychology Syndrome" *(1)*, which I had printed out. The topic of this article was how the gut and the psyche influence one another.

This article made me realise how harmful pathogenic gut bacteria can be. Their toxins can not only destroy the gut wall but also pass into the bloodstream and cause severe functional disorders and brain damage. These toxins are also believed to be responsible for autism spectrum disorder.

It was also very likely that Luca's anxiety was at least partly caused by certain gut bacteria and their toxic metabolic by-products. Autoimmune diseases are associated with these toxins as well. Luca had good reason to fear being poisoned, as this was indeed happening to him. However, the source of his contamination was not outside his body but in his gut, where resident microbes produced it. And technically speaking, the content of the intestines is actually outside the body through which the digestive tract runs like a tube.

When Dr Morrin entered the waiting room and called Luca up, he was surprised when only I approached him. I told him Luca was suffering from another flare-up and sleeping almost all day. He said that this was "very bad" and that I had to put an end to this. His comment almost sounded like a moral judgement to me. Did he not understand that Luca was utterly exhausted? He discussed Luca's blood test results with me, which had been "normal" when he was tested before Christmas. At least then, he had not been anaemic, meaning he had not lost any occult blood.

I wanted to talk with Dr Morrin about Luca's diet and my assumption that the unfavourable composition of his gut bacteria was the root cause of his colitis symptoms. Dr Morrin was not in the least prepared to go deeper into the topic. I explained my concern that I might not have been cautious enough with the diet. Certainly, he meant well when he answered that I had not made any mistakes. He said that Luca's illness had nothing to do with his food. "There are so many people who eat far unhealthier than Luca, and they also don't have colitis," was his explanation.

I was prepared for much, but to hear a trite

generalisation like this out of a doctor's mouth shocked me. We were talking here specifically about Luca and the effects that certain foods might have on *his* organism. This is referred to as "bio-individuality". I also touched upon Luca's contamination phobia and explained to Dr Morrin that I was deeply convinced that Luca's fearful thoughts contributed to developing his gut symptoms.

I also told him that the Department for Child and Adolescent Mental Health was no longer looking after Luca because his case was not considered "severe enough". Another reason was that we had not accepted that Luca should take psychopharmaceuticals. Dr Morrin promised to refer Luca to a psychologist again. He shared our view that drugs were not suitable for Luca's case. He told me it could be months until Luca would get an appointment, though, as the demand for this service was extremely high. I had read that one-third of Irish adolescents were suffering from mental problems. In some cases, youths in suicidal distress had to wait over a year for psychological or psychiatric therapy. The treatment with addictive psychopharmaceuticals was widely used as this was cheaper than talk therapy.

At the end of my visit, for which Dr Morrin had at least taken a lot of time, I placed Dr Campbell-McBride's article "Gut and Psychology Syndrome" on his desk. "Maybe you will find the time to read this article," I told him. Somehow the name "Dr Andrew Wakefield", mentioned in the article, jumped out at him. At the end of the 1990s, this gastroenterologist observed that most autistic children also suffer from an inflammation of the gut ("autistic enterocolitis"). I had no idea who he was. But Dr Morrin reacted extremely annoyed and started complaining that this man had maintained a connection between the triple measles, mumps, rubella vaccination and autism. Dr Morrin noted that he had been responsible for a decline in vaccinations in England and Northern Ireland at the time.

After this unsatisfactory visit to our doctor, I returned home disappointedly. I couldn't understand why Dr Morrin was not more open to our attempts to truly heal Luca's gut. Even if therapy with a specific diet was new ground for him, what prevented him from broadening his mind and professional horizon? Did our therapy approach not evoke his curiosity in the slightest bit?

Most professionals are permanently under pressure to obtain further training. And what about physicians? I had read it was widespread that the pharmaceutical industry sponsored additional training options for doctors. That makes it very unlikely that a nutritional approach for the prevention or treatment of disease is on the agenda.

Despite my dissatisfaction with Dr Morrin, I knew how hard it would be to find another doctor to meet my expectations. I decided to visit Dr Morrin only for Luca's blood tests in the future, which were due every four weeks. Anything else I would take into my own hands. Deep inside, Luca and I knew we were doing the right thing.

The following day, Luca didn't have to sleep during the daytime. He also didn't have any bowel movements. Gradually, our whole situation became more normal and relaxed again. The flare-up had lasted three challenging weeks.

A big success of my intensive internet research was discovering a press release from the Seattle Children's Hospital dated 28th December 2016. The headline was: "Novel Diet Therapy Helps Children with Crohn's Disease and Ulcerative Colitis Reach Remission". At Seattle Children's Hospital, the gastroenterologist Dr David Suskind conducted a small study with 12 paediatric patients. These patients followed the SCD for twelve weeks and received no additional medication to treat their active Crohn's or ulcerative colitis symptoms. At the end of the study period, eight out of ten patients who had finished the trial showed significant improvement in their symptoms. Remission had been achieved from the dietary treatment alone.

According to this article, in most clinics, inflammatory bowel disease treatment is limited to medications that suppress the immune system. However, the underlying issue, the patient's microbiome, must be addressed. "Doctors believe that IBD happens because something goes wrong between a child's genetic make-up, their immune system and their microbiome. In most people, the bacteria in the digestive tract are harmless. Although in some cases, the microbiome goes awry and causes a person's immune system to attack the bowel. It's still unknown why this happens," was the explanation given of the causes of Crohn's disease and ulcerative colitis. Dr Suskind pointed out that at the same time, it was necessary to acknowledge that each person's disease was unique, just as each person was unique.

As opposed to the dogma of conventional medicine, this study proved that diet had a powerful impact on inflammatory bowel disease. This study was the first of its kind and also showed that the SCD was safe and effective. Up to then, there had only been anecdotal evidence. "SCD is another tool in our tool belt to help treat these patients. It may not be the best treatment option for everyone, but it is an effective treatment for those who wish to try a dietary therapy *(2)*," says Dr Suskind.

Gradually – and even if only in very small steps – the SCD seems to get the recognition it would have been entitled to for over half a century because it does indeed work. Numerous case reports of patients who could achieve permanent remission from the diet alone prove this. In medicine, these case reports are referred to as "anecdotes", which has always irritated me. Outside the context of medicine, an anecdote is defined as a short humorous narration which records a strange event or a characteristic remark. These "anecdotes" are often played down and not taken seriously in conventional medicine. Anecdotal evidence may not be reliable on its own. However, it shouldn't be disregarded outright.

Medicine students are trained to only give attention to studies that adhere to the "gold standard". Only scientific data collected within a double-blind, randomised, placebo-controlled trial and then published in a prestigious scientific journal falls into this category. *(3)*

In his book "Wunder wirken Wunder" (wonders work wonders), which made it to the bestseller list of the German weekly "Der Spiegel", Dr med Eckhart von Hirschhausen stated: "The more individuals take part in the study, the more reliable is the result. Many miracle cures refer to highly impressive case reports, which are, however, not very well documented. And, as always, in a good story, you find embellishment and exaggeration *(4)*."

In principle, there is nothing wrong with having a sceptic attitude like this. However, extensive studies are costly and financed mainly by the pharmaceutical industry or sponsored by large corporations. As there is no money to be made with the SCD, insufficient funds are available for more extensive studies. And even Dr Suskind's small trial may not fulfil the "gold standard". Nevertheless, physicians should be more open regarding the SCD so that this diet and its effects can be further examined. In addition, one should always take a critical look at any scientific study, even if it does fulfil the gold standard because as soon as studies are motivated by personal or economic interests, distortions and manipulations of the study results are likely. That applies especially to studies commissioned by the vaccination or pharmaceutical industry.

In any case, I was thrilled with Dr Suskind's study. I would lay the press release on Dr Morrin's desk on our next visit. His claim that diet doesn't matter concerning IBD was in no way true!

Luca was feeling good again and had found back into his old rhythm. Also, his bowel movements were normal again. Everything was going fine, and I hoped it would stay that way. I was so happy to have the diet we had been following for circa two and a half months by then. And this is what Luca's daily menu looked like: Breakfast: Waffles (prepared with almond flour), steamed pear and apple slices and homemade SCD yoghurt. Throughout the day: Chicken soup, beef burger with cooked carrots or schnitzel with oven-baked vegetables or chicken breast with a mix of cooked carrots and pumpkin or pancakes (made from coconut flour) with SCD yoghurt and baked banana or cod with cooked courgettes.

1ˢᵗ February – St. Brigid's Day – The Beginning of Spring in Ireland

Diary-Entry:

Luca continued with his outdoor football training. He set himself the goal that his left (weak) foot would be as good as his right one by the end of the year. Although the training conditions could hardly be any worse – with a flooded, muddy meadow as a football pitch combined with heavy winds, rain and sleet – Luca won't let anything defeat him. He is entirely focused on his goal of becoming a professional football player. His passion resembles a flame that shines deep inside and constantly pushes him further. Nothing can stop him, not even his colitis. His motivation has no limits, and he knows exactly why he wants to become healthy again. And I will ensure that no one talks him into believing this is impossible.

I had brought myself to see my doctor, which I rarely do. As it was an extremely challenging time and because I was very tense and stressed, I felt I should also look after my own health. Of course, I informed my doctor about my worries regarding Luca's health. The more I told her about our situation, the less I could suppress my tears. My blood pressure was higher than optimal, which was certainly caused by my emotional state. My doctor warmly recommended that I make time for myself daily for physical activity and things I enjoy doing.

She was right. I had completely neglected my own needs. She advised me to get an appointment for a full blood count and to see her again for the results. I tried to find out her attitude toward dietary therapy for colitis. I also hinted that her colleague, Dr Morrin, did not seem to take the SCD seriously. She avoided a response. All she said was that the patient's safety always had priority. (By prescribing the drugs that are part of the standard medical treatment, doctors also make sure in the first place that they protect themselves.)

However, she told me about a local doctor, whom I knew by sight, who had suffered from severe colitis and was facing an imperative operation on her colon eleven years ago. She discovered the blood group diet of the American physician and natural healer, Dr Peter d'Adamo, and tried it out. Her results with implementing the diet spared her from the operation, and she has since been back to health. I appreciated this information greatly, as it nourished my belief that a dietary change can have a healing effect. I also found it reassuring that some doctors treated their colitis with a dietary approach. I looked up the blood group diet and found out that with regard to Luca's blood type (which is blood group 0), it was very similar to "our" diet. (Further information on the blood group diet is available in the appendix.)

On the following day, I was back in the

same joint practice. This time, however, I accompanied Luca, who had an appointment with Dr Morrin. While waiting, I asked myself why I still had not switched Luca over to my doctor and why we had remained loyal to Dr Morrin all along. However, during our visit, he was very friendly with Luca. He had sons of Luca's age who played football, too. Dr Morrin was also a great fan and liked to talk with Luca about current events from the world of football. It was moving how he treated Luca, and even thinking about changing doctors gave me a bad conscience.

Dr Morrin took Luca's blood sample himself instead of leaving it to the nurses. He was careful and gentle. A poster with a nostalgic painted image hung over the examination couch on which Luca was lying. It showed a friendly, almost fatherly-looking doctor and a little boy holding his teddy bear and standing in front of him. The doctor did not examine the boy but his teddy with a stethoscope. I know Dr Morrin has a demanding and stressful daily work routine, and I appreciate his dedication. I understand that many doctors feel drained and burned out because the conveyor belt medicine they have to practise in the conventional healthcare model has very little to do with why they became a doctor.

Luca was quite fond of Dr Morrin, which is essential for the doctor-patient relationship. However, I didn't feel that Dr Morrin could really help us. Before we left, I handed him the press release of the children's hospital in Seattle and said: "I have finally found a study proving the efficacy of the SCD." I hoped that from now on, Dr Morrin would take the diet and me more seriously.

It was the beginning of February. We had overcome Luca's low, and the mood barometer was improving again. Luca had cleared out his room, had decorated it differently and was very proud of it. He hung up his old FC-Barcelona and Germany jerseys, which were far too small for him now. Besides, numerous posters with his biggest football icons adorned the walls of his room. Neymar and Messi belonged to them, the latter life-sized over Luca's bed. It was unmistakable Luca's room, an expression of his personality and his creative talent. He felt cosy in his "den", and I had the impression that maybe it was only then that he had fully settled back in again. He seemed happy and balanced now that he could continue his training. All of this contributed significantly to his healing process.

On the internet, I came upon Jill Carnahan's website, where I read about the body's self-healing abilities. She is an American holistic doctor practising body-mind-medicine who believes that the root cause of many illnesses is in our minds. She thinks that nothing manifests in our body unless there is a mental pattern correlating to it. According to her, the law of life is the law of belief.

Therefore she advises that we should not say or believe in things that will harm or hurt us. Instead, we should use our thoughts to inspire us and others and to heal our bodies. She believes that our worries and fears may disturb not only the normal rhythm of our heart but also that of other organs.

For this reason, we should feed our subconscious with thoughts that lead to harmony, health, love and peace. That would enable our bodily functions to return to normal again. I cited a kind of prayer to Luca, which I liked a lot.

"My body and all its organs were created by infinite Divine intelligence, and it knows how to heal me. Its wisdom fashioned all my organs, tissues, muscles, and bones. This infinite healing presence within me is now transforming every atom of my body, making me whole and perfect. I give thanks to the Creator for the healing that I know is taking place now. This is the work of the creative intelligence within me given to me by God (5)."
(Dr. Jill Carnahan)

An absolute highlight in Luca's otherwise relatively uneventful daily routine was the arrival of his beautiful rosary, which he had ordered from nuns in Colorado Springs (USA). He had found the address of the "Sisters of Carmelite", who make rosaries and other religious jewellery upon the customer's special request online. The precious-looking rosary was made of black onyx beads, chain links and unique details from sterling silver. I wanted to thank the sisters for this wonderful work by email. I told them that the rosary was for my 16-year-old son and had a very special meaning for him as he was recovering from a severe illness. They answered me immediately. They also found that Luca had designed a particularly beautiful and tasteful piece. They said they would pray for Luca. It moved me deeply, and this friendly correspondence made us all happy.

On that day, Luca had trained for many hours. At night he lay in his bed with a feeling of satisfaction. Before going to sleep, he read an old football magazine that had fallen into his hands during his clearout. He fell asleep with his rosary around his neck, which he had worn for the whole day and which was much more for him than just a piece of jewellery. He had set out to find support on a spiritual level.

Meanwhile, my online research continued. I wanted to know whether an autoimmune condition could be stopped or even reversed. Everything I had learnt about it so far contradicted this hope of mine. Inflammatory Bowel Disease is classified as an autoimmune disease. The role of our immune system is to fight against anything that is "not self" and to protect what is "self". However, in the case of an autoimmune disease, the immune response is directed against the cells of our own body and can attack and destroy tissue and even whole organs.

I came across Dr Alessio Fasano's studies about gluten and the protein zonulin responsible for opening the intercellular tight junctions. In his scientific paper titled "Zonulin and Its Regulation of Intestinal Barrier Function: The Biological Door to Inflammation, Autoimmunity and Cancer", he wrote that autoimmune conditions (both intestinal and extra-intestinal), inflammatory and neoplastic disorders can occur "when the finely tuned zonulin pathway is deregulated in genetically susceptible individuals *(6)*." This new paradigm subverts the traditional theories that underlie the development of these conditions. It suggests these processes can be arrested if the interplay between genes and environmental triggers is prevented. And this can be achieved if the zonulin-dependent intestinal barrier function competency can be re-established.

Even if all of this sounded unfamiliar to me initially, was it different to what Luca and I were working on, namely to "heal and seal the gut", as Dr Natasha Campbell-McBride calls it in her book "Gut and Psychology Syndrome"? I had become curious, so I tried to learn more about this topic: In 2000, the worldwide recognised gastroenterologist Dr Alessio Fasano and his team discovered the molecule "zonulin", which regulates intestinal permeability. Until the 1980s, scientists had been convinced that the individual intestinal cells were "cemented" to each other and that nothing could pass in between them. Then Japanese scientists discovered spacings or "doors" between these cells, which were mostly closed. It had been unknown which signal was responsible for opening and closing these "tight junctions" for a long time.

Under normal circumstances, only fully digested molecules such as amino acids or monosaccharides (single sugars, glucose) can be absorbed through the gastrointestinal mucosal barrier. On the other hand, harmful substances, bacteria or toxins cannot pass through a healthy gut wall. For a long time, it had been a mystery how gluten, the environmental trigger for celiac disease, could pass through the intestinal wall and come into contact with the immune system. Fasano's starting point was that in celiac disease, there has to be an interplay between three factors: Number one is that the patient must have a specific genetic make-up to have an autoimmune response. Number two is that there is an environmental trigger for the autoimmune reaction to occur. And the third factor is that a signal exists responsible for opening the tight junctions to make an interplay between the first two factors possible in the first place. Dr Fasano found an answer to this mystery by discovering the molecule zonulin.

The gastrointestinal tract's epithelial cells (the top cellular layer of a membrane or skin) release zonulin in response to two major stimuli. The first trigger is the colonisation of the small intestine with bacteria (known as small intestine bacterial overgrowth or SIBO), which should not be present in this area but in the colon. As a reaction to the release of large amounts of zonulin, the tight junctions open, increasing intestinal permeability. As a result, water flows into the "lumen", the inner space of the intestine, which is normally filled with digested food or excrement. The water flushes out the bacteria and their toxins, leading to diarrhoea. The second stimulus is gluten, more precisely gliadin. When gliadin comes in contact with the epithelial cells, this also leads to the release of zonulin, which applies to every individual. Besides gluten, all kinds of other undesired substances can now pass through the gut wall.

The tight junctions of healthy individuals remain open for a short time only, and their immune system tidies up the damage without them noticing. People with celiac disease, however, produce far more zonulin, and their intercellular junctions stay open much longer. For this reason, there is an excessive flow of gluten and other harmful substances through the gastrointestinal mucosal barrier. And on the other side of the tight junctions, an immune system is waiting, which is not tuned to do its job right. Therefore, it reacts with an immune response that attacks the body's own cells and tissues. With celiac disease, the villi become blunted and destroyed, but other organs or tissues can also be affected. Patients with celiac disease must avoid gluten altogether. Some people feel much better if they stay away from gluten, even if they are not celiac. Their immune system also reacts to gluten, which leads to inflammation. These individuals are gluten sensitive.

Predicting flare-ups in IBD patients is possible by looking at their intestinal permeability. Patients with increased intestinal permeability, correlating with upregulated zonulin levels, are more likely to have another flare-up within the next few months.

If it is known what causes the breach of the intestinal barrier, it is possible to remove the trigger. If it is gluten, as in celiac disease or in gluten sensitivity, it is necessary to remove gluten. If the causes are bacterial overgrowth or dysbiosis, it is required to treat and fix this problem. Dr Fasano explains: "Either you treat the symptom [...] or you treat the cause. If you know the cause, you remove the cause, so it will go away that way *(7)*."

All this sounded as if we were on the right path. Could it be possible to go back again and correct where everything took its course? Could this become our road back to health? Luca did not ingest gluten anymore, even though Dr Morrin believed he had no problem with it. We had stopped feeding certain bacteria which stimulate the release of zonulin, and in this way, we were reducing them. And we did our best to nourish

Luca's intestinal cells with all the good things necessary for their regeneration.

Dr Morrin rang to inform me that Luca's blood values were all excellent. His inflammation markers were down, his liver and kidney values were well, and Luca was not anaemic. This information made us all very happy. Luca could discontinue the Salofalk rectal enemas he had used for the past month. We hoped he would not need them again. However, he continued to take the granules.

On the internet, I read that gut bacteria release highly toxic substances when they die, thus causing inflammation in the intestine. Maybe Luca's last flare-up had indeed been caused by eliminating more significant amounts of pathogenic bacteria, which we were no longer feeding. I would have loved to discuss my hypothesis with Dr Morrin, but unfortunately, he was not the right dialogue partner. Instead, Alex had to listen already at the breakfast table to my new findings about everything to do with colitis.

Luca's good form continued. He started eating cheddar and cashew nuts as a snack again because he had returned to training daily and needed a lot of energy. Luca felt very balanced and was in a great mood. One indicator was that he even took it with serenity when "his" team, FC Barcelona, lost in the Champions League against Paris Saint-Germain FC on 14th February.

However, the night following the match and the day after, he again felt a tearing abdominal pain. The beginning of his last flare-up was 40 days ago. We were alarmed. In the afternoon, Luca felt alright again, but he preferred to cancel his training in consideration of his gut health. The following day, he felt queasy, and in the evening, he complained again about the tearing abdominal pain and pain in his flanks. We held our breath and hoped this was not the start of another flare-up. The next day, Luca had more bowel movements but no diarrhoea. We hoped his intestines would overcome the crisis without the return of bloody diarrhoea. If it stayed away, it could mean that Luca's immune system was learning to handle more minor attacks without overreacting immediately. At least, this was my hypothesis.

Luca and I discussed matters of faith. He was convinced that he would become completely healthy again and could fulfil his plans and ambitions regarding playing football. I replied I was very proud of him and that everything would be well in the end. The next day was better. Luca was hardly in pain and only had two bowel movements. His stool was a bit soft, but everything was still in the green area. We hoped he was over the worst. For me, this would have been an indicator that Luca could reverse his disease.

I regretted that Luca and I had another argument that day. The reason for it was his contamination phobia. A few days ago, Luca finished his cleaning jobs by wiping all light switches and doorknobs and approved our house as being safe again. But now the whole misery started all over again. The fear of a new flare-up caused his feeling of security to collapse, and in his head, the red alert state was on. We had discussions up to the point of exhaustion. None of my arguments could change his firm belief that small traces of the toxic chemicals from school were present everywhere in our house and that these would be harmful to him if he were exposed to them daily. He was convinced that the "poison" would pass through the openings in his leaky gut and enter his bloodstream.

He told me that seven months ago when the bloody diarrhoea occurred for the first time, he was sure that the chemicals from the school had caused his intestinal bleeding and that he would have to die from it. He had not told me about it for days to spare me from the worry and pain. But after some time, he could no longer bear his fear alone. How much he must have suffered then. I was very shocked to hear that and felt terribly sorry for him. His fear had followed him until the colonoscopy in November as his flare-ups had reoccurred. He was relieved when he finally got his diagnosis because at least he knew this was not a fatal illness.

However, despite all my empathy, sometimes his compulsive behaviour made me angry. When I could not get through to Luca with my reasoning, he appeared to me like a stubborn child. There were moments when I just had to break free. Then I jumped on my bike as if bitten by a tarantula, and I pedalled as hard as I could to release my frustration. I didn't care whether it was raining or the wind was beating into my face or both, as long as I had an outlet for my frustration and could clear my head. Afterwards, I could see again that Luca was not a stubborn child but mentally and physically very ill.

I assumed that Luca's fear of death had caused his immune system to get completely out of balance. If you constantly think you are being poisoned, you will pass this message onto your body. Luca's immune cells also had to believe this at some point and reacted accordingly. Interestingly, poisoning with heavy metals can lead to colitis, an inflammation of the colon's mucosa. I had to help Luca get a grip on his anxiety disorder so his gut could heal, but how?

The following day began for Luca with painful pressure on his entire abdomen. Shortly after a bowel movement, he had to go to the toilet again. He had to pass a small amount of stool, and then hot blood flowed out of his body. Over the day, he had a few more bowel movements with small amounts of blood. His stool was still formed, but it appeared like being whisked (fermented rather than digested).

On this day, Luca ate a lot of chicken soup,

scrambled eggs, SCD jelly, yoghurt and chicken breast with vegetables. I also made ginger tea for him, which he drank over the day. We didn't want to reintroduce the Salofalk rectal foam again, as we hoped this flare-up would also fade away without this medication. If Luca were better the next day, it would have been his mildest flare-up, and we would have regarded this as a good sign.

Again, we were thinking about Elaine Gottschall's note that several relapses were likely during the first year on the SCD. In another source, I read more about the hypothesis that die-off reactions in bacteria strains could occur when you deprive them of their nutrition. That happens when their host makes dietary changes. As different strains of bacteria need specific foods, it is possible to selectively remove the nutrition of particular strains and influence the bacterial population in the digestive tract. However, before these bacteria are killed off, they become highly nasty and produce increased amounts of toxins, leading to inflammatory reactions in the intestine. If this theory was correct, we could see this flare-up as a good sign because it meant harmful bacteria said their goodbye.

The next day, Luca's bloody stools continued. In the daytime, he slept in an armchair in the living room and had at least seven hours of rest between his visits to the toilet. He hardly had any pain. I rang Dr Morrin, and we decided Luca should use the rectal foam again. I asked him how Luca's blood values could be so good only recently, and just a short time later, the inflammation was back again. Dr Morrin explained there was always low-grade inflammation which the medication kept in check. He reckoned it had been too early to discontinue the Salofalk enema.

Luca was a brave patient who wasn't pitying himself. This evening I wrote in my diary about how much I loved him. As in his childhood, he was still "my sweet little pet". Luca decided to reduce the amount of manuka honey he ate for its anti-inflammatory effect to one teaspoon daily. If he were infected with Candida albicans, at least he was not feeding this fungus with the food it flourished on.

I had read that this yeast fungus was present in the mouth and the digestive tract of 40 to 60 per cent of all US-Americans. Candida loves sugar and refined carbohydrates, and these are the food components that dominate our Western diets. Like ivy, which clings to the wall of a building and gradually destroys the construction, this fungus holds on to the gut wall. It eliminates the integrity of the intestinal mucosal layer (aka "leaky gut"). As a result, nutrition particles which are not fully digested can enter the bloodstream through the gut wall, which has lost its barrier function. The immune system recognises these particles as foreign and attacks them, which can lead to the development of food allergies, food intolerances and autoimmunity. If the integrity of the intestinal wall can be restored, these intolerances disappear in most cases.

Many doctors still refuse to acknowledge the existence of leaky gut syndrome. I once asked Dr Morrin if Candida albicans could be partly responsible for Luca's gut inflammation. All he replied in a know-all manner was: "Oh, don't go down that avenue now." Yet an infection with Candida would also have explained why Luca reacted slightly allergic to mould, why he always had a coated tongue and why his nose was congested all the time.

Luca also forewent cashew nuts for a while. Maybe they were too rough for his intestines. We introduced high-quality fish oil, which has an anti-inflammatory effect and a positive influence on the psyche.

An unexpected visitor provided some excitement in the evening of the following day. In the darkness, a yellow tit flew into our house. It fluttered back and forth in the living room and the kitchen, and we were worried that it could fly against the roof windows and get hurt. We opened the roof lights, but whenever the bird appeared to fly outside, it decided not to. It took us a while to understand that the little creature did not want to fly out because it could not see in the darkness.

Luca had the idea to turn off all the lights in the kitchen and switch on the light in the hall instead so that the bird would fly in this direction. That would enable us to guide it out of the house. At the same time, we had to pay attention that our cat didn't take advantage of the situation. In the end, we could solve this small challenge.

This visit had distracted us a little from Luca's new flare-up and did us all well. However, it also had its price, as Luca panicked the following morning. During our rescue mission the previous night, we used a torch in the kitchen and touched other objects and furniture. Luca refused to have his breakfast. He said he had to clean the kitchen first because the torch could be contaminated.

I freaked out completely. Not a discussion about the "poisonous" chemicals from the school again! In no time at all, I was dressed and off on my bike. When I returned after about an hour, I was soaking wet and blown through by the wind. In the meantime, Luca had made his breakfast and was back to normal again. I had also gained some distance. In the afternoon, I tried to find out more about obsessive-compulsive disorder online. As Luca could not count on support from a psychotherapist, I had to take over this role as well.

I found an article about the German TV-estate agent Hanka Rackwitz, a contamination phobia sufferer, who spends seven hours daily cleaning her apartment, only goes shopping with gloves, only buys shrink-wrapped foodstuff and only pays with her credit card to not have to touch any money. Her anxiety and compulsive behaviour determined her whole life, and I asked myself how this woman could function. I read out the article to Luca. He was also shocked about how much the phobia determined the patient's life. Luca said he would have only a few more things to clean. He promised that after this, it would be the end of it. I replied that he certainly had better things to do than cleaning all day. I was curious about how things would develop.

In the following days, Luca only had two to three bowel movements daily, which was all right. However, he also still passed varying amounts of blood. By now, it was Friday, our "salmon day" and the culinary highlight of the week. Shortly before dinner, Luca had to go to the toilet again. We were all looking forward to our meal, which I was just about to serve. Luca came to the table with a worried face. His stool had been covered with bloody mucus again. I talked to him and succeeded in calming him. I didn't want this delicious meal we wanted to enjoy together to be spoilt like this.

Luca's illness threw a shadow on our entire life. There wasn't a single morning when I didn't wake up without thinking of Luca's colitis immediately. After dinner, Alex and I watched a BBC music documentary that I found so interesting that I could switch off Luca's illness for a little while. It was after midnight when Luca finally went to sleep. It was the first night he didn't have a bowel movement straight after applying the rectal foam. We were glad because we assumed this medication would be more effective if it stayed inside his colon.

In the following days, I looked deeper into the GAPS diet, which Dr Natasha Campbell-McBride developed. Her diet is based on the SCD, and she has successfully treated her autistic son with it. I found out that a naturopath and nutritionist near us also had a GAPS qualification and experience in treating colitis.

It felt good to know that he could support us if need be, even though we didn't have the financial resources for treatment outside the conventional medical system. Since the start of Luca's flare-up, ten days had passed. His stool became firmer again and only contained tiny traces of blood. As his flare-up seemed to near its end, Luca dedicated himself again to his cleaning chores. That probably stressed him so much that he had several bloody bowel movements again. It was difficult for Luca to believe in his healing progress. Being unable to clean and create a safety zone for him depressed him.

I visited my doctor to discuss my blood test results with her. All my blood counts were good, and my blood pressure was normal again. However, I broke into tears when we started talking about Luca. I lost control completely, and all my suffering burst out of me. As a mother, I had always tried to do everything "right". I had guarded Luca with my life, not only after his birth but also during my pregnancy. So many mothers weren't doing half as much as me for their children. Why was it that their children were healthy and Luca was so ill? How had I deserved this? Again, I felt like the victim of a massive injustice.

My GP patiently listened to me sobbing and pouring my heart out. When I was finished, she said: "Unfortunately, this is not how life works, and life isn't necessarily fair either." She was concerned about my health if I didn't learn to cope better with Luca's illness. She asked me if I was interested in receiving counselling. Surely this would help me. She could arrange an appointment for me if I wanted to. Without hesitating, I accepted her suggestion.

On the following day, Luca felt a little better. Just a tiny amount of blood was left in his stool, and he only had one bowel movement in the morning. His appetite was good. His diet comprised scrambled eggs, bone broth, chicken breast, salmon, steamed carrots, and steamed butternut squash. He had enough energy to return to his cleaning job. Luca and I decided to start with the GAPS diet and to order Natasha Campbell-McBride's book "Gut and Psychology Syndrome" online. At midnight, Luca came into our bedroom and informed us that his stool was normal again. Of course, the three of us were relieved, but I was utterly exhausted.

On the following day, Luca's flare-up seemed to be over. His pain was gone, and his stool was finally back to normal. He continued with the cleaning. I suggested he say "never mind" to himself whenever he felt pressured to clean something. Then he should just let it be and try to increase saying this to himself by one more time every day. I considered this a good idea, but I wondered if Luca could put it into practice. I wanted to put an end to his obsession to prevent it from becoming a permanent habit. I presented Luca with an ultimatum. I would go on strike in the kitchen if he wasn't finished by the weekend. He promised to try.

The next day, Luca was in a bad mood. It was incredibly grey outside with persistent rain. For the past two weeks, Luca had been unable to train. The flare-up had lasted the entire second half of February, and in the meantime, it was March. I told Luca it was perfectly all right to be fed up. He decided to clean his "highly contaminated" shoes. These were the ones his classmate had poured "toxic" chemicals on. In addition, Luca had to clean all the other shoes that were standing on the shoe rack. About ten pairs of shoes must have stood in the rain after this operation.

Alex freaked out when he saw his soaking-wet Sunday shoes standing outside. As far as I was concerned, I didn't care any more about what was happening to our shoes. I was only hoping that Luca's "therapy" would help him somehow. On the one side, I found it positive that he confronted himself with the "poison" and did not swallow down his anxiety or repress his fear. But then again, I doubted his cleaning obsession would ever end. However, with every "contaminated" object he cleaned, Luca seemed to become more relaxed because, in his view, the amount of poison in our house decreased.

Luca and I talked a lot about his contamination phobia. He told me he had had it since Christmas 2014, over two years ago. That was a long time. I remembered that back then, he had also suffered from a globus sensation in his throat for months. For me, it was clear now that the chronic stress, combined with his unfavourable diet, had led to his colitis. Even if a genetic predisposition played a role in developing his symptoms, environmental factors were the trigger. In a study by the American physician Dr Michael Bailey, I found my assumption confirmed that stress could suppress the immune system or cause it to be overreactive.

Luca's fear was like a ping-pong ball that jumped forward and backwards along the gut-immune-brain axes, and in doing so, it developed an uncontrollable dynamic. As soon as Luca's gut symptoms returned, his contamination phobia also worsened. His brain caused the release of stress hormones, fuelling the inflammation in his gut even more. And this again increased his anxiety. Sometimes the fear of a new flare-up was already enough to trigger it. At least, this is the impression that we got. One morning Luca told me that on the previous evening, he had thought about the "poison", and shortly after, he had abdominal pain.

My mood barometer rose when I discovered on the internet that autoimmune conditions could disappear spontaneously. I wished so much that this would also be true for Luca and that the story of his illness would have a happy end. A newspaper article a friend had brought along also gave us new hope. It was about the Irishman, Ian Lacey, who had been diagnosed with ulcerative colitis (UC) at 17. His doctors had told him he would be on medication for the rest of his life. When Lacey was 30 and told his doctor that he was planning a bicycle trip from Alaska to Argentina, he was shocked and advised him against it.

Nevertheless, Lacey took on the challenge and pushed himself to his limits. On the 27,369 kilometres long route, he felt better and better every day and better than ever before. He started reducing his medication. The article ended with the sentence: "Meanwhile, Ian has suffered no further bouts of UC, and he no longer needs medication *(8)*."

Mind and Soul

"By changing the way we think, we change our life."
(Henry David Thoreau, 1817–1862)

The 6th of March marked the start of a new week and the beginning of a transformation of my whole thinking. I had my first prescribed consultation appointment. Mairead, a delicate Irishwoman who must have been far in her sixties, welcomed me into her sparsely equipped workroom, where two big armchairs faced each other. We sat down, and she asked me what had led me to her. I told her about Luca's illness, our experience with our doctors and the diet, our ups and downs and the burdens connected with it all. I gave her a brief insight into our personal history so she could better understand our situation.

When Luca was thirteen, we relocated from Ireland to Germany, as we felt that this would be better for Luca's further development. That was in the summer of 2013. Luca and I had stayed with my mother in Germany the previous summer. During this time, Luca had the opportunity to test his future school for a few weeks. In the beginning, even only the thought of it frightened him. Luca only knew his rural school in Ireland with less than 50 pupils. It was tiny compared to the enormous

German "learning factory" with almost 2000 students. Nonetheless, he settled in quickly and liked it.

When we returned to Germany in 2013, intending to stay longer, Luca could return to his trial school class of the previous year. He already knew the other pupils and didn't find it hard to settle in. Although, in the beginning, Luca had problems with German orthography, he kept up with the curriculum surprisingly well. Because of his football skills, he was very popular with the other boys and could form friendships quickly. Luca enjoyed his morning rides to school on the school bus and loved that he could reach everything in our small town by bike. It gave him a degree of freedom and independence he had never experienced before, as in Ireland, he always depended on being driven everywhere.

There were four football clubs in the town. Luca picked one and became a member. In addition, there were amateur football fields, and he could practice football on the road in front of my mother's house. The weather, at least compared to Ireland, was outstandingly good. Luca was pleased about his new living situation. Finally, he had all the conditions which supported him in his intention to become a footballer. I knew that this was everything he had ever wanted. It was his place of origin, and finally, he had arrived home.

Alex and I had undertaken this step for

Luca. We were optimistic that we could gain a foothold in our home country again. We still had our old circle of friends, and reviving our existing relationships didn't take much effort. Alex had a job in prospect, which we had relied upon. Maybe we had been too trusting, as a short time after our arrival, we had to find out that the promised vacancy didn't even exist. That was the beginning of the end. Both of us had no work and lived from our savings. We tried to find a job, but this was far more difficult than we had imagined. We had been abroad too long to know how the wind blew in Germany.

We belonged to the "50-plus-generation", and the prospects of finding an adequate job were not good. Besides our frustration about the job situation, Alex was unhappy about living with my mother in her home. We had been too naïve. We had the best intentions and wanted to create a better future for Luca, but our venture was deemed to fail.

Alex decided to return to Ireland by the end of the year. I could understand him, but I wanted Luca to finish his school year and stay until the following summer. I had succeeded in landing a few jobs as a translator, but they were poorly paid. If we hadn't been able to live with my mother, Luca and I wouldn't have been able to manage economically. It was a sad situation, especially for Luca, who enjoyed his new life but knew that his happy time would soon end. He suppressed his painful thoughts about having to return to Ireland as long as possible.

Up to the end of our stay, I had tried to find a well-paid job. I had well-maintained professional qualifications, but I realised that the labour market was no longer interested in me due to my age. In addition, my CV had too many "gaps". Consequently, Luca and I returned to Ireland after the summer holidays, where Alex had already enrolled Luca in his new school.

Luca's new learning environment was a significant change for him, but he seemed to handle it positively and confidently. We were surprised at how well he appeared to deal with everything. It took about three months until we realised that appearances were deceptive. That was in the autumn of 2014. More and more frequently, Luca asked the school secretary to ring us because he wanted to be collected from school early. He felt unwell and weak and was afraid he would faint. It was only much later that he told us that his new classmates, who had respected him initially, took advantage of his weakness and started to bully him. His former classmate and yearlong "friend" also participated in the bullying activities. He stabbed Luca in the back to move up a rung in the existing pecking order.

After the Christmas break, I could hardly make Luca go to school. He had developed a globus sensation in his throat and chewed for ages on every bite before he could swallow it. He was afraid to suffocate from it. Luca could hardly eat breakfast, and it got later every morning before he could get to school. For being late, his first school break was cancelled. It meant that he was also not allowed to eat anything. On one occasion, he secretly took a bite from a cereal bar because he felt dizzy. The teacher in charge ordered him to spit out his food immediately.

Luca had told Dr Morrin that he had no energy and always needed to eat something. By now, he no longer left home without bringing food, as he was always afraid to faint. I asked Dr Morrin to write a letter to the school principal stating that Luca must always have the opportunity to eat something. He wrote a short note which said that Luca has to suck glucose between the lessons now and then.

Dr Morrin had no answer to our question about the reasons for Luca's problems. He referred him to a psychotherapist. Initially, I also believed that Luca's symptoms must have psychological causes. I supposed he didn't want to go to his new school and tried to make him go by putting him under enormous pressure. Luca had always been an outstanding and ambitious pupil. For me, it was like the end of the world when he suddenly stopped cooperating and functioning the way I wanted him to. Of course, I was also worried about his future.

At some point, his gut symptoms started. Each morning shortly before he had to go to school, he got diarrhoea. In Dr Morrin's opinion, I was too soft with Luca and had to toughen him up. So, in the beginning, I sent Luca to school despite his frequent diarrhoea. As time progressed, I came to realise that Luca simply couldn't continue like this any longer. His illness had been the only solution for him to get out of the dilemma between the expectations he had to fulfil and his own needs.

"The greatest mistake in the treatment of diseases is that there are physicians for the body and physicians for the soul, although the two cannot be separated."
(Plato, approx. 427–347 BC)

In retrospect, I believe that Luca was already heading towards his colitis then. However, I am convinced that it could have been prevented. Physical, psychological, emotional and social factors were involved in Luca's disease development and interacted with each other. The attempt to treat Luca's problem only on a psychological level while ignoring all his physical symptoms was medical malpractice.

Many symptoms pointed in the direction that Luca suffered from gluten sensitivity or gluten intolerance; hence, they were symptoms of toxicity. That would also explain why Luca felt so much better just a few days after introducing the SCD, which is a truly gluten-free diet. There are a lot of diagnostic testing procedures available which provide information about gluten and food intolerances, a dysfunctional microbiome (dysbiosis, Candida albicans, and parasites), pancreatic insufficiency (enzyme deficiency) or increased permeability of the mucosa (leaky gut). These saliva, blood, or stool tests go beyond what most health insurances are prepared to cover and are not considered by most doctors. We would have been prepared to pay for essential examinations out of our pocket. Already then, Dr Morrin should have examined what the matter with Luca's gut was. Or he should have referred him to a competent gastroenterologist.

Instead, he interpreted Luca's symptoms as mentally based and sent him to a psychologist. In this way, he got rid of a patient to whom he couldn't offer solutions. Psychological support was also important for Luca, but not as the only treatment option. It was not a matter of "either-or" but of "as-well-as". Luca had a damaged gut *and* a hurt soul. He couldn't find the right words for his fears, emotional suffering and inner conflicts. It would have been our duty and that of Luca's GP to interpret Luca's physical signals and to put them into words. Together we could have talked about what troubled him.

Luca was very much afraid of the physical symptoms he was experiencing. He didn't know where the pounding in his temples was coming from and what caused his abdominal pain, diarrhoea, permanent exhaustion and dizziness. Besides, he only wanted to become a footballer and fully identified with this goal. Every day it seemed less realistic to reach it, and his sorrow about this caused him further stress. He had had enough of being regarded as someone who was only making his symptoms up. Sometimes he wished the others could *see* that he was indeed ill. A year later, his wish came true. No one can ignore bloody diarrhoea. The barrel had overflowed. Too many disease-causing factors had affected him for much too long. His body could no longer find back into equilibrium or a harmonic flow.

After our return to Ireland, the disappointment about our shipwreck in Germany was gnawing at me. It hurt me that Luca was forced to give up his happy time and new life again. As time passed, I tried to arrange myself with it and gain a foothold in Ireland again. But as further flare-ups tormented Luca repeatedly, the repressed disappointment rose to the surface again and manifested as rumination: Why had our plans not worked out? What should we have done differently? Why did Luca have to suffer so much? Why were we all in this lousy situation where I couldn't even work? The looping thoughts in my head never ceased. I was blaming myself, although I had tried everything. I felt guilty about Luca's illness.

Mairead held herself back and only asked a few questions. Besides that, she just listened. Of course, I also had to cry. She pointed at a box of tissues lying on the ground next to me. I helped myself, thinking that many tears must flow in this room. At the end of my first appointment, I felt utterly exhausted. I had spoken almost for an hour. It wasn't hard for me to open up. It felt good to put it all into a story and, in doing so, to gain some distance. Through this, I could learn to handle our situation better instead of constantly getting overwhelmed by my emotions. We arranged another meeting for the coming Monday. I thanked Mairead for listening to me. I wasn't sure how our sessions would develop and what would come out of them, but I wanted to try them. I had nothing to lose.

The state of Luca's gut improved every day. He only had one daily bowel movement, and his stool was solid again. His diet changed little and comprised poultry, bone broth, cooked pumpkin, carrots or courgettes and scrambled eggs. Luca had not kept his promise to finish his cleaning by the weekend. And I had not put the consequences I had used as a threat into effect.

All the time, Luca's fear made him find new objects that could be contaminated. One day, he focused on two big wicker baskets filled with bags and backpacks. One backpack was Luca's former school bag, and this was his primary concern. In

Luca's eyes, it had also contaminated all the other contents of the baskets and the baskets themselves. In the evening twilight, he carried everything to the edge of the stream that flows through our land. He wanted to clean everything in the stream. Some bags he weighed down with stones so he could leave them overnight without them being washed away. It drizzled and had already turned dark when he returned to the house, where he warmed his cold, stiff hands in front of the fire. He said he would be finished by the end of the coming week as there wasn't much left to clean.

The evening held a highlight ready for Luca. The Champions League was broadcast on TV: the return match between FC Barcelona and Paris Saint-Germain FC. FC Barca had to achieve a difference of five goals to move on and make up for the defeat of the first match. It was somewhat unrealistic but not impossible for the team, which took pride in being "more than a team". Indeed Messi and his team could decide the match with a result of 6:0 at Camp Nou. It was a top performance. Luca floated in happiness; it was late before he went to sleep.

The following morning surprised us with a cloudless blue sky. The sun was shining onto our breakfast table, and we soaked up the light and the warmth. We had done with no sunshine for much too long. We let Luca have a sleep-in. When he joined us later, we enthusiastically discussed the outstanding match result of the previous night. I explained to Luca that it showed the importance of having the right mental attitude. I told him he could overcome his fear if he only wanted it enough. If he could release his inner blockages, this would allow the energy in his body to flow more freely. His self-healing abilities could then make him well again.

As I didn't feel understood by our doctor, I tried to find advice and inspiration from doctors on the internet who I felt were more on the same wavelength as me. Mostly I landed with American physicians who were practitioners of Functional Medicine. My online research led me to the YouTube channel of the American chiropractor and holistic physician Dr John Bergman. When I watched his videos, I understood a few things concerning the interests of "Big Pharma". I felt confirmed in my assumption that the pharmaceutical industry could not truly be interested in healing a patient. In particular, this applies to patients with "chronic diseases" as they are lifelong clients.

One good example is proton pump inhibitors (PPIs) which are prescribed for heartburn and acid reflux to reduce the stomach acid of people affected by these symptoms. However, Dr Bergman explains that in most cases, acid reflux is not caused by too much but by too little stomach acid. Even if these medications may lead to short-term relief of symptoms, they aggravate the underlying problem. In addition, antacids or acid blockers, as they are also called, can lead to several severe adverse effects. Some patients take them for decades, particularly because some products are available over the counter. (In the Irish Lidl, I saw them next to the sweets. How appropriate!)

The function of stomach acid is not only the breakdown of protein. It also kills bacteria and pathogens we ingest with our foods or drinks and prevents them from moving further into our intestines. A lack of stomach acid increases the risk of bacterial gut infections and also causes abnormal colonisation of the intestinal mucosa. IBD patients often have too little stomach acid, which can lead to dysbiosis, leaky gut and autoimmune diseases.

Physicians should know it better, but they prescribe these medications, which are so popular that the pharmaceutical industry makes gigantic sums with them. In the US alone, 13 billion dollars are spent on acid blockers yearly. *(1)* Billions for a wrong kind of treatment, which does not address the cause of the symptoms, makes patients dependent on drugs and causes other conditions like cardiovascular disease. I had never been a friend of medications, but this lesson was a real eye-opener for me.

In this video, Dr Bergman also talked about a 17-year-old ulcerative colitis patient who – in her short life until then – had received 40 vaccinations and had an unhealthy diet. Unhealthy, in her case, means too many refined carbohydrates, too much sugar, and too many unhealthy fats (which negatively impact the ratio of omega-6 to omega-3 fatty acids in the body, fuelling inflammatory processes), genetically engineered foods and nutrition contaminated with glyphosate.

Dr Bergman treated the young woman by adjusting her spine, which led to an improvement in the energy flow in her body. He also made her change her eating habits, meaning she started eating "real food" prepared from organic produce. These interventions reduced her body's inflammation and made her symptoms disappear gradually. Dr Bergman is convinced that the human body is designed to repair itself and keep itself healthy. All it needs is a normal nervous system function, regular exercise, a healthy diet, sufficient sleep and relaxation, prayer and meditation (healing begins in the mind).

Information like this was essential to me. Without it, supporting Luca on his path back to health would have been even more challenging. We needed hope instead of the negative brainwashing saying there was no cure for Luca's disease. I felt the conviction that Luca would become well again, growing stronger within me. In my colitis diary, I wrote: *"Luca will be healthy again. It is only a question of time. Even if there are setbacks, he will have a full recovery!"* Nothing and nobody would dissuade me from that.

However, this did not change the fact that Luca looked extremely stressed because his obsession drove him to clean "contaminated" objects. I had the feeling that his mental state got worse rather than better. The more he cleaned, the more he became aware that it would take a very long time to tick off everything from the to-do list in his head. Besides, Alex and I sometimes unintentionally destroyed the results of Luca's work by touching things he had already cleaned with our "contaminated" hands. It meant that he had to clean them again.

Luca cleaned all the pens and other writing utensils, spectacles, remote controls, and everything we used daily. Before I could prepare any food for him in the kitchen, he had to make his round and this several times per day. Luca cleaned all the handles of cupboards and drawers, the knobs of the cooker, the water tap, etc. He wouldn't eat anything if he couldn't be sure that his food wasn't contaminated.

I kept telling Luca over and over again that there was nothing in our house to be afraid of and that Alex and I weren't worried about any contamination, either. Nonetheless, I accommodated Luca by constantly washing my hands just to make no "mistakes". I felt so much under pressure that I submitted to his control. I knew that this wasn't really helpful and that, instead, the opposite was the case.

I didn't want Luca to eat any food that he considered harmful to him. I was afraid that feeling unsafe could trigger another flare-up. It is known that for some people, the fear of harming themselves or suffering physical pain is already enough to develop physical symptoms. That is referred to as the "nocebo-effect", in which the power of the mind negatively impacts the body.

Luca feared that the effects of the "poison" might manifest only years later. That made everything even more complicated. Had he been afraid of the immediate consequences, I might have been able to convince him to take the risk and see what would happen. If nothing had happened, he could have convinced himself that his anxiety was unfounded, and maybe he could have let it go.

Sometimes I watched him when he was sitting in his favourite armchair in the living room. His face was distorted with pain, his body was completely tensed up, and his hands were clenched into a fist. He was probably thinking about everything he still had to do – a bottomless pit. Or, because of a "mistake" that Alex or I had made, he realised he had to clean all over again. When I watched him sitting there like this, I suffered with him. I was unsure if he could overcome this problem without the support of a psychotherapist. But then again, I hoped that with all his cleaning, he might feel that he had removed enough contamination to feel safe again and relax.

The constant stress was toxic for Luca; there could be no doubt about it. I was glad he was not afraid of bacteria because he would never have been able to get these guys under control. He was also not worried about natural dirt. It was the unpredictability of chemical substances that he feared. And principally, this fear is not unjustified. Rather, the opposite is the case, as we have left our children with a planet that resembles a toxic minefield. The attempt to live healthily has become like a ridge walk.

According to the US health authority CDC (Centers for Disease Control and Prevention), 25 per cent of all children in the USA suffer from a chronic condition. Some experts even speak of 50 per cent. Nowadays, young children are already diagnosed with diseases that just a few decades ago only occurred in older people. That is shocking, and for a reasonably intelligent and sensitive young individual, our present reality can indeed be scary.

If you want to be and stay healthy today, you have to make choices outside the mainstream, be it regarding your diet or lifestyle. That is not easy, demands a lot of awareness and should also not become another stress factor in your life. It used to be normal to live healthily because people were not surrounded by as much junk as today (not just regarding our diet, but also our mental food).

You didn't have to think so much about whether something was healthy as there weren't as many traps you could fall into.

In our modern time, however, you could start questioning everything you consume. Beginning with the water you drink (filtered water from the tap [which can still contain chlorine, lead or other chemicals], water from plastic bottles [contaminated with BPA, also less environmentally friendly] or water from glass bottles [expensive, not available everywhere and because of the weight, you might need a car to transport it], continuing with the consumption of fish (a source of healthy omega-3-essential fatty acids, but also contaminated with harmful heavy metals and other environmental toxins) or the use of smartphones (the best option would be not to use them at all, but this does not help much if the next transmission mast is just around the corner). Nowadays, it is hardly possible to live an entirely healthy life. You have to be ready for compromises. And then again, you should not worry too much, as stress is also a disease-causing factor.

Coming back to Luca, I could observe how his anxiety went off the rails; in parallel, this was also happening to his immune system. Not just the psyche and the immune system, but all the systems in our body constantly communicate and interact. Almost everything in the body is connected with everything else. Our body, mind, and soul cannot be separated.

I had my second appointment with Mairead. We talked about Luca's contamination phobia and his colitis. In her opinion, I had to learn to develop more inner distance. First, I was harming myself if I identified too much with Luca's suffering. And second, Luca had to feel I was calm and in control. Having a worried expression on my face all the time certainly wouldn't contribute to his healing. That made sense to me. I told Mairead about what I had discovered in a book by the Ayurvedic physician, meditation teacher and bestselling author Deepak Chopra: that genes could be turned on and off. *(2)* This was new to me. Up to this point, I had believed that our genetic make-up was unchangeable and that we couldn't influence it.

I explained to Mairead why this new insight was so important to me because it meant that the alleged "genetic cause" of colitis was only a partial truth. Could it be that we didn't simply have to put up with Luca's bad luck in the genetic lottery? Were our genes not our fate, as it was always claimed, and were this fatalistic attitude and genetic nihilism simply wrong? And how substantiated was the alleged hopelessness of inflammatory bowel disease, after all?

"Genetics" was a catchword for Mairead to play a podcast for me. It was an interview with the renowned American stem cell researcher and pioneer in epigenetics, Dr Bruce Lipton. His following statement made a lasting impression on me. He explained that, in most cases, an individual's health did not mirror their genes but how environmental factors influenced them. Genes directly would cause less than one per cent of all diseases. To 99 per cent, it depended on how we reacted to the world.

We have control over our genes and are not their victims. The American scientist and physician Dr Dean Ornish proved this in his often-cited study *(3)*, in which he made prostate cancer patients change their diet and lifestyle in a health-promoting way. Within 90 days, the patients' switches for the activity of over 500 genes could be altered. Many of these changes in genetic expression suppress biological processes, which play a role in the formation of tumours *(4)*.

How is this possible? Only two per cent of our genetic material (DNA) consists of genes which are blueprints or building instructions for proteins. When scientists discovered this, they prematurely labelled the remaining material as "junk DNA". However, there is no waste in nature, and everything has its function. Later, scientists discovered that this non-coding DNA contained over 4 million "switches", which can turn genes on or off. That only makes sense, as the genome for our complex human organism has only 19,000 genes, not more than that of a microscopically small worm with only about 1000 cells.

The enormous number of gene switches reacts to epigenetic mechanisms (activities "above the genes"), making it possible for our 19,000 blueprints to code for over 100,000 different protein molecules in our body. Epigenetic factors influence how genes are read and "printed" without changing their DNA sequence. The alterations of the functioning of genes don't have to be valid for an individual's whole lifespan. Epigenetic mechanisms are responsible for the ongoing dialogue between our genome and our environment and ensure our adaptability to environmental signals. Our diet, our lifestyle, the emotions we have or the stress we are experiencing are all part of these environmental factors.

Indeed our genetic heritage only plays a relatively minor role in developing a disease. Nonetheless, many people are experiencing their genes as ticking time bombs and are afraid they will act against them at some point. They are waiting to develop their mother's or father's cancer. The pharmaceutical industry and the media also fuel this fear.

After an hour with Mairead, my mindfulness coach, I was filled with new insights, inspiration, and hope. Luca, Alex and I faced a difficult stage full of stones and boulders on our way. However, with joint forces, we could get there and heal Luca.

Maybe it was also necessary to heal us as a family. Over the last few years, the three of us had experienced a lot of disappointment and hurt, and each of us had tried to deal with it individually. Maybe Luca had become a "symptom carrier" in the superordinate organism that a family represents.

Back at home, I told Luca about Bruce Lipton. We decided to watch some of his YouTube videos in which he talked about the influence of subconscious negative beliefs on our behaviour. What I found even more interesting was that our beliefs can also influence the expression of our genes, physiology and health. Lipton stated that our subconscious mind governs 95 per cent of our behaviour. The biggest part of our beliefs – often the ones that can lead to self-sabotage – are downloaded to our subconscious mind before the age of six without the control of our critical thinking. In our later lives, most of the time, we switch to autopilot and hand over the control to our subconscious mind. When our conscious thoughts, desires, and goals meet with the negative beliefs imprinted in our subconscious, this leads to disease-causing tension and stress. Lipton also mentioned methods to influence what had been programmed into our subconscious mind, for example, "EFT tapping".

Luca was impressed by this approximately 70-year-old American who came across as an approachable, young at heart, very likeable guy and not at all as a serious or even snobbish professor. We got aware that the endless tape that I kept playing in my head and also Luca's contamination phobia were only thoughts, like trains on which we kept jumping instead of just letting them pass by. Bruce Lipton became my new "guru" who opened up a new, fascinating world to me with his book "Biology of Belief". Luca and Alex often made fun of me when I couldn't wait and already had to tell them at the breakfast table about my new knowledge. Then they called me Professor Dr "Hase" (hare), the latter being my nickname.

Alex and I discussed that we had to find an alternative to the conventional medication that Luca was taking. I was worried about their adverse effects and discovered that it was possible to treat colitis homoeopathically. We did not have the financial means for alternative treatment as I had been unable to work as a translator for the past months. Anyhow, we felt that we owed it to Luca to protect him from the possible adverse effects of his medications. We had never mentioned them to him. However, he had often expressed his doubts about whether his drugs were helping him at all.

The following day offered a welcomed change to us. Our long-standing friends Maureen and Kevin, both in their late seventies, had taken a trip from Dublin to Abbeytown to see us. We were all looking forward to an opportunity to catch up again. We arranged to meet at Luca's hairdresser.

Luca hadn't been out anywhere for a long time and wanted to use the opportunity to get a haircut. Luca's hairdresser asked him if he was on any medication. He had noticed immediately that Luca's hair was very brittle and that he had hair loss at the temples. Luca also had severe skin irritations on his face. I am not talking about the usual pimples that teenagers have but inflammation in deeper layers of the skin. These kinds of spots hurt and did not come to the surface. They were more like small ulcers, bleeding when opened but didn't discharge any puss.

After Luca's appointment, we went to the closest coffee shop with our friends. Kevin and Luca chatted about football, a shared interest which had given them plenty to talk about over the past years. A small collection of books about nutrition, which was lying on a windowsill, attracted my attention. A book titled "Gut" fell into my hands, and it turned out to be the English translation of Giulia Enders' bestseller "Darm mit Charme".

A friend living in France had already told me about this book, which was making the rounds there. The gut and particularly its population had become an important topic everywhere except for the consulting rooms of Luca's physicians. It is hard to believe, but none of Luca's doctors had ever mentioned the term "microbiome" or anything linked to it.

More about

The Gut Flora

The gut flora (also: gut microbiome) is part of the flora which populates our entire body. It predominantly consists of bacteria, fungi and viruses. The more diverse and balanced it is, the better our overall health and mental stability are. Up to 1,400 different species of microbes are known, which can potentially populate our gut. In a healthy person, the number of microbes is limited, and they are controlled by friendly gut bacteria. "Civilised" humans host between 150 and 200 different types of bacteria. More than double the amount of healthy bacterial strains can be found in the intestines of people living in alignment with their ancient traditions. Everybody has a unique microbiome shaped by one's personal history, diet and lifestyle.

Approximately 100 billion bacteria populate the gut surface with a weight of about two kilograms. One-half of our stools consist of bacteria, and one gram of faeces contains more germs than the number of people living on earth. We have ten times more microbes in our bodies than human cells. We may find this consideration rather bizarre, but this makes us only ten per cent human.

The beneficial microorganisms themselves and their metabolic products are essential for our well-being. They produce hormones, messenger substances (neurotransmitters), proteins and antioxidants. Bacteria also can influence our genes. As revealed by the human genome project, a human has less than 20,000 genes. That is only one-fifth of the number of genes scientists had expected for the complex human organism. The microbes that populate our gut, skin and mucous membranes make up for the genetic information we don't have.

Until about ten years ago, relatively little was known about the gut flora as only two per cent of the gut bacteria can be cultivated under laboratory conditions. The remaining bacteria are anaerobic, which means they die when they come in contact with oxygen. Therefore microbiologists never took notice of them, let alone examined them. However, since 2007, also anaerobic bacteria can be studied with the help of genetic screening. Today, "dysbiosis" (disturbances in the composition of the intestinal flora) is thought to be at least partly responsible for a broad spectrum of diseases. These include autoimmune diseases such as inflammatory bowel disease or type 1 diabetes, depression, anxiety, dementia, overweight, allergies and certain skin conditions.

Experts refer to the entirety of our microbiota as an independent organ with an intelligence of its own. Each type of bacteria has its characteristic features and abilities, and together with the human being, they form a complex network. Some bacterial strains work together hand in hand. The microbes communicate and interact between them and with us. They take over tasks that the human organism cannot perform by itself. In return, we provide them with food and accommodation. When everything is going well, both parties profit from it. We call this relationship "symbiosis".

If our gut were sterile, it would be unlikely that we could survive. Our digestive tract is the largest contact area with the outside world and is constantly exposed to microorganisms, chemical substances and toxins. We can only master this situation with the support of our friendly gut microbes, such as bifidobacteria or lactobacteria, which live on the intestinal mucous membrane and keep it intact and healthy. They provide a physical barrier and natural protection against invaders, undigested food, toxins and parasites. All these substances and unbeneficial microorganisms can harm our digestive tract and cause chronic inflammation in the gut wall. Friendly gut bacteria keep harmful and opportunistic ones in check and ensure they do not gain the upper hand.

In the case of chronic inflammatory bowel disease, pathogenic bacteria are present in the gut mucosa and even in the gut cells. The protective shield provided by friendly bacteria is broken, enabling pathogenic bacteria to reach the vulnerable gut wall. Without healthy gut flora, the gut is unprotected and malnourished, making the gut wall even more vulnerable.

A well-balanced gut flora supplies the intestinal mucosa cells with energy and nutrients. An estimated 60 to 70 per cent of the energy the gut epithelium requires stems from bacterial activity.

Beneficial bacteria can produce substances with antibiotic, fungicidal or antiviral effects. They produce interferon and other substances that destroy the membranes of viruses and harmful bacteria and stimulate the immune system to react appropriately to invaders. In addition, "good" bacteria produce organic acids, which lower the pH value near the gut wall to a level of 4.0 to 5.0. This acidic environment makes it difficult for pathogenic, harmful bacteria to settle there and thrive, as they prefer a higher pH value.

Pathogenic microbes produce a large amount of very potent toxins. In addition, there are also the toxins we take in with our food. Our friendly gut bacteria can neutralise a significant number of these toxic substances. They can also inactivate histamine and chelate (remove) heavy metals and other toxins.

Friendly bacteria can even protect us against cancer. Their cell walls can absorb and inactivate carcinogenic substances. In addition, they suppress hyperplastic processes in the gut, the basis of cancer formation. *(1)*

I flipped through Giulia Enders' book, which appeared informative and quirky. I showed Maureen the funny illustrations, but I don't know if it was her type of thing. Although having lived in Ireland for decades, the Englishwoman had remained very British in certain things, and the intestinal tract and its products were not her preferred table talk. After the coffee, we accompanied our friends through Abbeytown to the Arts Gallery, where they wanted to look at paintings by Jack Yeats. We said goodbye and drove back home.

For Luca, it had been a good day. He said that his life had felt a bit more "normal" after a long time. He hardly had any social contacts and spent most of his time at home. The next day was the 17th of March, St. Patrick's Day, the Irish national holiday. It rained from morning until evening, and many regional parades had to be cancelled. Luca was exhausted and slept long. I noticed he was very thoughtful for the whole day. On the following day, his mood was very low. He figured out when his next flare-up would be due. That, of course, was in no way beneficial for his recovery.

Inspired by Natasha Campbell-McBride's highly recommendable book "Gut and Psychology Syndrome", in which she also precisely explains the GAPS diet, I tried to make sauerkraut for the first time in my life. The author explains fermented foods used to be part of the diet in every culture and still are in places. The lactic acid bacteria therein are essential for maintaining a healthy gut microbiome. However, in our Western diet, fermentation has been replaced by the use of multiple stabilisers, and this is detrimental to the gut flora.

While working on the sauerkraut, I remembered an old big earthenware sauerkraut pot serving my mother as a flowerpot. It has a capacity of at least 20 litres, and my long-deceased grandmother used to ferment her sauerkraut in it. How much I would have loved to get her advice now. I pressed the cut and salted cabbage into a mason jar and hoped I would successfully culture loads of gut-friendly bacteria.

We felt that we were somehow not getting anywhere. We wanted to switch to Natasha Campbell-McBride's GAPS diet because we hoped to achieve better results. The GAPS diet is based on the SCD but is stricter and gives more precise instructions. The diet comprises various phases, and in the introduction phase, patients are only allowed to eat bone broth. Luca had been on the SCD for four months already, so we needed to figure out where to start with the GAPS diet.

The answer soon came by itself. Only two days later, Luca had another flare-up. It had announced itself beforehand by Luca feeling "somehow different" and suffering from hot flushes. Besides, the skin of his face looked extremely irritated. However, Luca didn't feel as groggy and hardly had any pain. When the bloody diarrhoea returned, we were much more composed than we had been on the occurrence of the other flare-ups.

Diary-Entry on the 19th of March:
A long journey lies ahead of us before Luca's full recovery, but we will tackle the challenges together and learn a lot on our way.

Because of the new flare-up, we decided to start with the GAPS diet from its beginning and strictly comply with the specified schedule. Of course, we knew one could not force anything, but we were determined to have success with the diet. So we began with step 1 of the introduction phase.

In the beginning, the new flare-up dragged on for six days relatively moderately. Luca was disappointed that he could not train, but he felt well enough to edit the video material he had filmed before and to publish new football videos on his YouTube channel. The editing was easy for him, and he had fun doing it.

Luca had hardly any pain and a maximum of three bowel movements which contained relatively small blood amounts. He also didn't feel as weak as during the other flare-ups. His gut may have already healed to some degree and therefore was more robust.

Indeed, one could also have claimed that it was thanks to Luca's medications that a more severe inflammation had been prevented. However, we doubted the efficacy of his drugs and asked ourselves if they didn't even hinder Luca's healing process. The medications didn't stop the flare-ups or make them any shorter. The intervals between the flare-ups were the same as they had been at the beginning of Luca's condition when he had not been on any medication. I wondered if the flare-ups followed some rhythm related to the bacteria's life of their own. Anyhow, sometimes we asked ourselves why Luca was taking the prescribed medications at all.

Again I spent considerable time at my laptop, searching for information that could help us further. By coincidence, I came across the sample chapter of the German book "Ein medizinischer Insider packt aus" (A medical insider tells the whole story). This narrative non-fiction was published under the pseudonym Prof Dr Peter Yoda. I decided to read the entire book. What I read about the practices of "Big Pharma" shocked me. Still, at the same time, I felt vindicated in what I already had assumed: The pharmaceutical industry or the medicinal system systematically intimidates patients to make them compliant. Hence, they take their medication, even if they have a number of adverse effects that are toxic to the body and lead to other diseases, which are also treated with drugs.

The American health documentary series "Betrayal: The Autoimmune Disease Solution They're Not Telling You" shook me, in which over 85 Functional Medicine experts discussed autoimmune diseases. Here Dr Peter Osborne claimed that, according to a study about the top causes of death in the United States, "medical error" was the third leading cause of death directly after heart disease and cancer. This study had been published in the prestigious "British Medical Journal". It was proven data and not something he had made up. Osborne asked if the use of prescription medication, the third leading cause of death in the US, did make any sense. In his opinion, depending on the pharmaceutical industry and conventional medicine was the wrong thing to do.

"From a business perspective, medicine is the only business to grow at an exponential rate despite failing miserably its customer. What other business can you think of other than government that has that track record?" so Osborne. "Any system that makes 100 billion Dollars annually that fails to lead their customers to some form of meaningful resolution has to re-evaluate their business model *(6)*," he continued.

According to Osborne, any intelligent individual can figure out that the conventional medical system is built on masking symptoms and, in the process of doing this, on creating new diseases with the drugs it uses. (In the US, it is not rare that patients take up to 20 different drugs.) "Autoimmune is notorious for this. For example, immune suppressive drugs that are used to treat lupus and arthritis, they cause cancer; it is very clear on the warning label. They cause cancer; they shut down the immune system. Is that a solution? Is that something we want to give 100 Billion Dollars a year to as a solution? *(7)*" says Osborne.

Again it became evident to me that we had to find an alternative to the conventional drugs that Luca was taking. I found studies about herbal remedies. *(8)* I came across an article about the efficacy of probiotics in treating ulcerative colitis. In scientific research, it could be proven that the probiotic Escherichia coli Nissle (Mutaflor by Ardeypharm) was effective in achieving and maintaining remission in patients with ulcerative colitis. In a comparative study, E. coli Nissle was proven to be as effective as mesalazine.

In more recent studies with the probiotic product VSL#3, a combination of eight different probiotics (Bifidobacterium breve, B. longum, B. infantis, Lactobacillus acidophilus, L. plantarum, L. paracasei, L. bulgaricus and streptococcus thermophilus), the efficacy of this preparation could also be confirmed. However, a sufficient dosage is necessary for probiotics to achieve the desired effect. *(9)*

Why had none of the doctors who treated Luca ever suggested using probiotics if they are not inferior to mesalazine and have no adverse effects (at least to my knowledge)? And how can it be that gastroenterologists do not advise their patients to take probiotics after a colonoscopy?

In her highly recommendable bestseller "Schlau mit Darm" (Clever with Gut), the German gut expert Dr Michaela Axt-Gadermann points out that building up the gut flora systematically after a therapeutic fasting cure is critical. At the start, you empty the bowels with the help of a laxative. Dr Axt-Gadermann explains that after a complete purge of the intestines, the diversity of the gut microbiome decreases drastically. The author characterises the new constellation of gut bacteria as "dangerous, to be more precise inflammatory". She states that after the purge, "different germs have a say, namely those present in inflammatory bowel disease or irritable bowel syndrome *(10)."*

She also points out that the regeneration of the gut flora should also be supported with probiotics and/or prebiotics after a colonoscopy. Before this examination, your bowels have to be completely emptied, and afterwards, they are especially susceptible to the uptake of pathogenic germs. *(11)* So why is it that after a colonoscopy, gastroenterologists do not take better care of their colitis patients who already have a damaged intestinal flora?

I have spoken to several individuals who had a colonoscopy in the context of a preventive check-up. None of them had been advised by their gastroenterologist to take probiotics after the procedure to regenerate their gut microbiome. Is this due to indifference or a lack of knowledge, or does it have to do with the fact that gastroenterologists cannot prescribe probiotics and hence do not earn any money from recommending them? Luca and I had often discussed that the best opportunity for implementing his diet, in combination with probiotic therapy, would have been immediately after his first colonoscopy. Unfortunately, we didn't know then what we know now.

Diary-Entry of the 25th of March 2017:

Just back from a walk with Rover: The sun was shining on my face and warmed my whole body. The soft ground gave in gently to each of my steps. Blue sky, the first yellow blossoms of daffodils, wild primroses and gorse. The first leaves are coming out. Birds' twittering, the sound from our stream and the waterfall up the mountain, the voices of bleating sheep in the distance. Despite my cold and Luca's ongoing flare-up, the feeling: Life is good, and everything will be fine. I accept that I will be responsible for Luca's diet for an indefinite time. If this leaves me time for anything else, I will gratefully receive it as a bonus.

I accept that Luca became ill. However, I do not see it as irreversible fate but as a signal of his body and a chance for him to truly heal. I am grateful for having the financial freedom to prepare healthy food for him and to help him. What would be a better way to show him how much I love him? Luca told me that as a young child, he remembered an incident from the time before his birth. He was looking down from above, watching me. He was talking to a circle of individuals and chose me as his mum. Even today, Luca has no doubts that this really happened. Maybe everything is the way it is supposed to be, and everything we experience has a deeper purpose. Tomorrow is Mother's Day. Today Luca is very low and depressed. Maybe I can give him a lift with my cheerful mood.

Farewell to the Medications

On Mother's Day, which fell on the 26th of March, I had a severe cold. However, I walked in the sun with Luca, and we talked a lot. Luca was fine and didn't feel any pain. His stool was more solid again, with hardly any blood in it. On the following night, Luca used the rectal enema. Straight afterwards, he felt a searing pain in his intestines, and then the bloody diarrhoea was back. The following day also began with bloody stool.

Luca told me about his suspicion that "the Salofalk" only worsened everything. Until then, I had mentioned nothing to Luca about the adverse effects of his medications, but now it was the time to talk openly about them. We looked up the effects of mesalazine (5-amino-salicylic acid) on the internet. That was the active substance in the granules Luca was taking orally and in the Salofalk enemas. One of the "side"-effects of mesalazine is BLOODY DIARRHOEA *(1)*. I couldn't believe my eyes. A medication causes exactly the symptoms for which you are taking it. I was flabbergasted. Luca was also shocked. He said: "Mama, is it possible that my medications keep destroying the healing progress that we are working on so hard? Maybe I would already be far better if I hadn't taken them at all."

I had learnt that non-steroidal anti-inflammatory drugs (NSAIDs) could destroy the balance of the gut flora and even attack the gut wall. Although mesalazine was structurally related to these medications, it didn't belong to the same category. Therefore, I couldn't really answer Luca's question. However, I was immediately thinking of the posts on the internet by patients who reported that they had been taking the standard repertory of medications for colitis (from mesalazine to steroids to immunosuppressive drugs) for the past fifteen years, but their condition continued getting worse. Was it possible that their medications were at least partly responsible for the decline of their health? Taken together with the fact that the root cause, namely their dysbiosis, leaky gut and other possible factors, hadn't been addressed in all these years?

This incident was the final trigger that, on the very same night, I rang the homoeopath I had already selected and arranged an appointment. He was also German and had been living in Ireland for many years. On the phone, I told him what I had found out about the "side" effects of Luca's medications and all he said was: "Does that surprise you?" – "Well," I replied, "of course, I knew that medications have side effects, but it is new to me they cause exactly those symptoms that they are supposed to alleviate. That is a sheer perpetuum mobile. What it means is that you will never get healthy again." It crossed my mind again that the global market for IBD medications was estimated to amount to 6.7 billion US dollars for 2017. *(2)*

I asked the homoeopath if he had experience in the treatment of colitis. He did, and he gave me hope that he could help Luca. A weight had been lifted off my shoulders. One more week and we would see him. I asked if Luca had to discontinue his drugs so he could be treated homoeopathically. I was relieved when the answer was "yes". First, Luca discontinued the Salofalk rectal foam. Three days later, on the 27th of March, he took the Pentasa granules for the last time.

Although I felt the medications had not benefitted Luca, I kept asking myself if we were doing the right thing during the first drug-free days. Now, I had to take responsibility for him, which initially frightened me. The pharmaceutical industry's strategy of intimidation had been successful. The feeling of insecurity that tormented me was not new to me. It had felt similar when I decided against specific vaccinations for Luca, such as the swine flu vaccination carried out in his primary school after a few sporadic cases in Ireland. In Luca's classroom, only two other parents besides us had decided against the vaccination for their children and had not given in to the fear-mongering.

Now I felt glad and proud that I hadn't let myself be guided by the majority then but had

followed my inner guide. And this time, it was also
the right decision. Deep inside myself, I knew that.
Luca also didn't want to take the medications any
longer, although initially, he was convinced they
would help him. Now he felt betrayed by his
doctors and the pharmaceutical industry.

I asked him if he had any other symptoms
that could be related to his medications. Luca
complained about back pain and pain when passing
water. (Kidney and liver damage are also listed as
possible side effects.) He had difficulty swallowing
and also pains in the chest area. He suffered from
sour burps or acid reflux. The acne on his face was
severe. Before his colitis, he sometimes had pimples
in the "t-area" (forehead, nose and chin), which had
disappeared. But instead of these, he had purple
skin inflammations deep under the surface of the
skin on his cheeks, temples, and both sides of his
chin. (Some of the inflammations caused
permanent scars, which will always remind him he
was stronger than his disease.) Sometimes he had
nosebleeds which had been unknown to him
before. In addition, he had pains in his legs, and his
toes were swollen and had a purple colour. When
he was wearing shoes, his swollen toes pressed
against each other, hurting for that reason. Also, his
hands and forearms had a purple skin tone at times.

We could find all of these symptoms on the
extremely long list of side effects. *(3)* Even now,
while writing them down, my breath is being taken

away. And Luca was supposed to take these medications for at least two years, if not for the rest of his life? Drugs with far more unwanted than desired effects, with the latter not even occurring?

"Open your medicine cabinet and count your medications! Read the side effects on the instruction leaflets of these pharmaceutical preparations! Regarding most medications, you accept being poisoned for their effect. These forms of poisoning manifest as 'side effects'. This expression is deceptive. For sure, it sounds better for yourself and the pharmaceutical industry to speak about side effects here rather than poisoning *(4),*" writes the alternative health practitioner and bestselling German author Uwe Karstädt in his book "Entgiften statt Vergiften" (detoxify instead of poisoning yourself) about side effects.

[**Important advice:** I would <u>explicitly</u> ask you not to take my account as a reason to discontinue your drugs by yourself, especially not from one day to the next. Principally, medication should be "tapered", which means slowly reduced following your doctor's advice. I am fully aware that very severe and even life-threatening complications can occur in the context of inflammatory bowel disease. I do not want to play down this fact at all and advise you always to put your safety or that of the patient first.]

Luca felt significantly better on his first

drug-free day than the previous one. He put this down to discontinuing his drugs and was happy about this step. We started with phase two of the GAPS diet. Early on the following morning, Luca came into our bedroom to tell Alex and me that his stool was much firmer. He said that he had slept very well, much better than in a long time. Then Luca went back to bed again. Shortly afterwards, he noticed a searing pain in the horizontal part of his colon. Luca had to go to the toilet urgently and passed some bloody mucus. Then he went back to sleep. He felt good for the rest of the day and had no pain. He had no bowel movement for the following 14 hours.

In the night, Luca suddenly felt this searing pain again and the urgency to pass stool. According to Luca's description, it felt as if something had burst in his gut. His stool was mushy, and at the end, it was followed by blood. It was the first time that I was seriously worried about Luca. Was it possible that some ulcer had burst in his intestines? And if so, what would that imply? Maybe we should bring him straight to the hospital? Perhaps he was in acute danger? – However, after his bowel movement Luca was feeling well again, and the pain had disappeared. With his hands, he could even put pressure on his abdomen without feeling any pain.

Luca noticed that the symptoms he had then felt different from those during his previous flare-ups. He asked himself if his momentary symptoms could have anything to do with his medications. I couldn't answer his question. I only hoped the homoeopathic treatment would help him because it simply couldn't go on like this.

The next day also started for Luca with diarrhoea containing small traces of blood. However, for the rest of the day, he had no symptoms at all. The inflammation on his face calmed down a little bit. I assumed that the state of his facial skin mirrored the state of his gut.

Luca was firmly convinced that the medications had harmed him and held up his healing process. I shared his opinion. Luca's body was already stressed enough. It couldn't deal with any additional stress from the drugs' chemicals.

Luca and I talked about his illness and how he saw it. On the internet, he had found a sentence suitable for his situation: "God gives the hardest battles to his strongest soldiers." Luca said that his disease was a challenge he had to master. When he succeeded, it would be his goal to inform other people about his experience to help them on their way back to health or to see that they don't get ill in the first place. People would listen to him if he succeeded in becoming a famous football player. I was very moved and proud of my son.

On the following day, the 31st of March 2017, Luca had firmer stool without any blood for the first time again. All in all, he had been feeling much better since he was off his medication. Was this just a coincidence? Luca told me it had been like a flash of insight that he had to stop his medication. He said it had felt the same way when he had found religion some time ago. "All of a sudden, I simply knew what I had to do", he said. "I was certain that it was due to the drugs that my last flare-up continued forever." I had often noticed that Luca had a very intensive body perception and a keen sense of what was happening inside him. He was also absolutely confident that he would return to health through the diet.

And this is how his menu for the day looked like: freshly pressed vegetable juice, scrambled eggs with SCD yoghurt, ginger tea, lamb casserole with carrots and pumpkin, poached salmon, cooked carrots and courgettes, peppermint tea, scrambled egg with yoghurt, manuka honey and omega-3-fish oil.

I had started preparing a tasty, freshly pressed juice from cabbage leaves, carrots and celery. Cabbage has a lot of beneficial properties, including an "anti-ulcer factor". It can alleviate or heal inflammations and ulcers in the gastrointestinal tract. The compound responsible for this is called L-glutamine. The American physician Dr Amy Myers refers to L-glutamine as the "number one ingredient for the repair of a leaky gut". *(5)*

While reading about the magic cure "cabbage", I remembered an incident from my childhood. Once, my grandmother had cured a deep and inflamed cut on my thumb, which had not healed well, with a poultice made from cabbage leaves. How sad it is that long-standing household remedies like this one, which have no side effects and are mostly very inexpensive, have been pushed aside by modern Western medicine and the pharmaceutical industry. It is about time we reclaim this valuable knowledge and use it again.

1st of April:

Early in the morning, Luca came into our bedroom to tell us that his stool was completely normal again. That was great news. However, he was worried for the whole day as he was feeling pain in his chest area, and he feared the drugs' side effects could cause it. I told him this was possible, but the symptoms would disappear. Luca's body started detoxing from the drugs he had been taking, as now his tongue had a green colour for days. The skin of his face was still looking stressed. On the positive side, he had a lot more energy. For the first time in weeks, he picked up a ball again. He was itching to restart his football training.

The Way Up

Luca was able to eat a more versatile diet now. It consisted of scrambled eggs with SCD yoghurt and banana, salmon, turkey breast, cooked carrots, courgettes and pumpkin, bone broth, a combination of cooked peppers, courgettes and aubergines, pancakes, chicken legs with carrots, meatballs made from minced meat and chicken breast with vegetables from the wok. When he felt like it, I also served him small amounts of the sauerkraut I had made. Up to then, he had only been allowed to have the juice.

Luca also started taking a probiotic food supplement. We used a product containing 14 different strains of live bacterial cultures. In her book mentioned above, Natasha Campbell-McBride advises increasing the dose gradually. We started with one capsule daily and increased the dose by one capsule every two to three days. Luca's full dose was six capsules corresponding to 12 billion live bacterial microorganisms. In addition to these, he also consumed fermented foods containing probiotics.

At the end of the first week of April, we had an appointment with our homoeopath, who spent over an hour on Luca's first anamnesis. We outlined what we believed was relevant to Luca's momentary overall state of health. There was no time pressure, and we could talk to a health practitioner who was listening to Luca's history and was trying to see the whole picture. As I am always eager to learn, I was curious to receive a short introduction to homoeopathy.

This medical system goes back to the German physician Samuel Hahnemann (1755–1843), who was not happy with the brutal treatment methods of his colleagues. In his view, disease symptoms showed the patient's struggle to overcome an illness. Rather than suppressing the symptoms, he found it much more sensible to stimulate the body's self-healing abilities. Homoeopathy is based on the principle of similarity: a substance that leads to specific symptoms in a healthy individual will cure similar or the same symptoms in a diseased person. The more you dilute and shake ("potentiate") a homoeopathic drug, the stronger and more profound the effect will be, provided it matches the patient's needs.

In Luca's particular case (as not every colitis patient receives the same remedy because homoeopathy is not a one-fits-all approach), our therapist chose the drug Lycopodium (club moss) and mixed a tincture from it. He explained to us how Luca had to dilute it further and how to take it. After finishing his remedy, Luca should wait a few days and then make contact again. If this were the appropriate remedy for Luca, we would not have to come back, at least not for his colitis. But perhaps Luca needed another remedy that suited him better. We were curious to find out what would happen.

On the following day, we started with the homoeopathic therapy. As we knew that this drug had no side effects, Luca felt safe when taking it. With the conventional medications, he had always felt an inner resistance which he had suppressed as he knew he "had to" take them. We were relieved that this pressure was gone. I swore to myself that I would only resort to conventional medications in the future if they were essential for my survival.

With each day, Luca felt better. Gradually his stool lost its grey colour, and very soon, it was no longer one of our conversation topics. Around the middle of the month, we had an appointment with Dr Morrin. He informed us about the results of Luca's blood test. Luca lacked a bit of folic acid and was slightly anaemic, but besides that, everything was fine. Before the last blood test, Luca had suffered from a very long flare-up which had reduced his red blood cells. We informed Dr Morrin that Luca had discontinued his prescribed drugs two weeks ago. We listed all the side effects which Luca had experienced. Dr Morrin did not say anything. I told him that Luca had started to take a probiotic preparation and showed him the package. In addition, I presented him with the study mentioned above about probiotics' efficacy in treating colitis. He took a glance at it. I asked him if he could prescribe probiotics to Luca. He said he couldn't because they were not considered drugs but labelled as dietary supplements.

Patients must pay for probiotics, which are scientifically proven to impact the microbiome positively. But drugs which are only effective in 30 to 50 per cent of IBD cases and have considerable side effects are covered by health insurance. These drugs are usually prescribed for a lifetime. The treatment of health conditions, which have arisen from their side effects, is also covered.

This regulation, which doesn't make any sense to me, isn't serving the patients but pharmaceutical companies. The pharmaceutical industry can only embrace the trend that an ever-increasing number of individuals suffer from unhealthy gut microbiomes forcing up the number of chronically ill patients. If probiotics were prescribed and thus more widely used, they could become a real competition to standard drugs.

With the correct selection and dosage of probiotics, it is possible to reduce inflammatory messengers and positively affect the immune system. "Microbes can change many switches in our body, and by doing so, they can influence important processes *(1)*," says Dr Axt-Gadermann. The rescue could come from the bacterial front, particularly in autoimmune diseases, as in these conditions, the gut flora can act as a warmonger or peacemaker. Probiotics don't only have a positive impact on the population of bacteria in the gut but also in other regions of the body, such as the nasal mucosa. From where they are located in the gut, specific probiotics can increase our stress resilience and even reduce our stress hormone levels. Dr Axt-Gadermann thinks that we will be increasingly less dependent on antibiotics and medications in the future. Instead, treating disease symptoms at their very roots with microorganisms will be possible.

This approach was also followed by the Russian Nobel laureate and immunologist Ilja Metschnikow (1845–1916). He studied the beneficial health effects of fermented milk products. He traced back the longevity of Bulgarian peasants to their regular consumption of yoghurt and the lactic acid bacteria contained therein. He regarded the species "Lactobacillus delbrueckii subsp. bulgaricus" as particularly helpful.

In our time, scientists can avail of a lot more sophisticated methods (for instance, the DNA sequencing of bacteria) to examine the effects of particular bacterial strains on the physiology and the health of a human being. Some probiotic bacteria can already be systematically deployed. However, scientists are far from knowing all the specific characteristics and abilities of each strain of our intestinal population.

It is still to be determined whether the perfect microbiome exists and what it is supposed to look like. However, what can be said with certainty is that a wide diversity of bacteria positively affects our overall health. A healthy diet can only have its full potential in cooperation with healthy gut flora. And our microbiome's composition can be influenced by how we feed our "bacteria zoo". Accordingly, Dr Axt-Gadermann says: "The state of the gut and its inhabitants is, above all, dependent on what we eat. The typical diet of the 21st century, with plenty of sugar, far too little dietary fibre and far too many ready-made meals and highly processed foods, does not promote friendly microbes at all. Our friendly gut bacteria are starving in front of our full plates *(2)*." Physicians are simply wrong when they tell their patients that chronic inflammatory bowel disease has nothing to do with their diet.

I didn't talk with Dr Morrin about Luca's diet any more. I also considered it better not to tell him about Luca's homoeopathic treatment. It was a pity as I knew there were clinics in India or Germany where modern Western medicine, homoeopathy and other traditional medical therapies coexist. Different therapeutical approaches don't have to compete with each other but can be used complementarily for the patient's well-being.

Easter 2017:
All of us abstained from Easter eggs and Easter bunnies made from chocolate. I boiled some eggs

and dyed them with plant colours. These kinds of Easter eggs were also a good alternative for Luca. As a starter, I made a "nest" from puréed avocados on which I placed two egg halves. Luca liked this idea. He told me that he had seen a TV advertisement for Lindt Easter bunnies without having the slightest cravings for chocolate. That was remarkable because there had been no Easter without the classic golden Easter bunny for as long as he could remember.

Luca was training every day on our property now. He was outdoors for three hours and felt good and energetic. For weeks, his footballs had been lying idle in his room, and his football boots were covered with delicate spider webs. Luca wanted to shoot at a proper-sized football goal the following day and asked us to drive him to "his" training pitch in the nearby village. I accompanied him and used the opportunity to take a long walk at the seaside. Afterwards, Luca continued his training at home. He was a real bundle of energy. I was delighted and grateful that Luca was in such good form again. It was the day before my birthday, and my only wish was his health.

On the 20th of April, Luca took the homoeopathic remedy for the last time. He felt great. His body supported him perfectly with his football training. He kept doing his left foot training to be able to play with both feet. Only a few professional football players have two equally good feet, and Luca wanted to become one of them. Luca had reached the full recommended dosage of probiotics at this time. He tolerated them well, and they didn't cause him any major flatulence.

As Luca was a little bit prone to constipation now, I followed Dr Campbell McBride's tip and prepared sour cream. It is made like SCD yoghurt, the only difference being that the milk is replaced by cream. The result is a kind of crème fraîche which is full of probiotics. As sour cream is fatter than yoghurt, it provides a rich and healthy energy source. In addition, it has a positive effect on the immune system and the nervous system. *(3)* It also acts as a gentle laxative and makes the stool smoother. Luca tried the sour cream immediately and stirred a few spoonfuls into his vegetables. He liked it very much, and ever since, sour cream has become a daily part of his diet.

With his vegetables, he ate the velvety, tender steak with which a good friend of our family had surprised him. "Before, it had been sweets, and now I am bringing you some steaks. I told the butcher I only want the best meat for you, and he cut it freshly," she said to Luca. I greatly appreciated how our friend adapted to Luca's new needs. The steaks were from Irish cattle allowed to graze on the land all year round. No wonder Luca tucked into his delicious meal with relish!

After a short digestion break, he continued

with his training. I watched him practising his "bin shots". He had placed a large square plastic bin in front of my flowerbed and was trying to kick the ball inside it from about twelve meters away. I reflected on how my perceptions and priorities had changed since the beginning of his illness. Before, I would have gone berserk if a ball had fallen into my flowerbed, destroying my plants. Now it just was not important to me any more. I was happy and grateful that Luca was well again and had the energy and motivation to train. Before getting angry about something, I asked myself if the reason for my anger would still be relevant in a few weeks, a few months or a year. If this was not the case, I tried to ignore the reason for my anger.

On that same evening, the sour cream showed its effect. After three days without any bowel movement, Luca was relieved that his digestion was running smoothly again. Luca told me that now he could feel his body being fuelled with new energy a short time after a meal. He hadn't experienced this feeling for a long time, and eating something hadn't really affected his energy levels.

Lacking energy isn't necessarily based on an insufficient intake of calories. It also makes a significant difference from which food sources these calories stem. It is also not entirely correct to say, "you are what you eat" because it is crucial that you can digest and absorb the nutrients you take in properly. In addition, the energy in the body also has to flow. Stress, negative beliefs or unprocessed grief can block energy flow, which can lead to disease symptoms.

1st of May:

Today is the first summery day. It is a delight to feel the sunshine on my skin after the seemingly never-ending winter. When I walked across our meadow with Rover this morning, the melody and lyrics of "Morning has broken like the first morning..." suddenly came into my mind. Even if it may sound cheesy, it simply was appropriate. The fluttering butterflies were having a race, the lambs on the adjacent field were calling their mums, the birds were chirping, and a cuckoo was calling. I quickly cleaned the chicken coop, and in return for the daily cleaning service, I was rewarded with three body-warm eggs lying in the nest. It was precisely the right amount for Luca's pancakes.

I would have loved to spend more time outside, but as usual, the kitchen was full of pots and pans, which needed washing up. I had to prepare yoghurt and finish the bone broth I had started to make. It did weigh me down a little bit that I had to spend most of the day in the kitchen again. I was thinking of the beach, which was only a few kilometres away, and of my bike standing idle in the shed. But I was so abundantly rewarded: Luca was feeling great. For about five weeks now, he had not been taking any medications and had been without any symptoms. Luca had the energy to train for hours, making him more than happy. He loved the food I prepared for him; his body could absorb and utilise the nutrients optimally.

At the Beach (the 8th of May):
There are hardly any clouds in the sky, and the sea is calm. In the distance, a woman and a man with a young child paddling on an air mattress in the ocean, screeching. I decide to walk to the end of the beach, which I have entirely to myself. I enjoy the gentle, rhythmic sound of the waves, the soft, cool breeze and the smell of the sea. On the way back, I take off my shoes and walk barefoot for the first time this year. The tide and the currents have left different traces on the sand, and while walking, I can feel the various structures and degrees of hardness of the ground under my feet. I take photos of the shades of blue and wonder when I will return to painting again and if I can reproduce these colours. I pick up a piece of sea glass which is turning into a worry stone in my fist. Two horsewomen are approaching me, galloping at first, then slowly reducing their speed. On the hazy horizon, the steep Slieve League cliffs slide into the water. The tide is coming in. I am enjoying the present moment, and I am happy that Luca can train on the other side of the dunes.

10th of May:

A powerful, almost cloudless day. I am sitting in a deckchair and close my eyes. I feel the pleasant warmth of the sun on my face. The cool air gently caresses my naked feet. I try not to think, just to feel and to listen: the variety of songs from the different birds, the humming of a bumblebee coming nearer and then moving away again, the cheerful clucking of our chickens, the engine noise of a tractor and the bark of a dog from a distance. A moment of inner peace and aware enjoyment. Just being there and knowing that life is good until Rover nudges me with his cold nose, and I start thinking about the dirty pots and pans waiting to be washed up. I hear Alex with the chainsaw in our small grove. He is making firewood for the stove, which must be fed on most evenings of the year, as days like this are rare and a real blessing.

I hear the rhythmic sound of a ball being juggled. Luca is training in football freestyling. It makes him happy to be able to make progress. His passion for football motivates him to become fit and healthy again.

Luca's gut is well, but the contamination phobia has him in its grip again this morning. The trigger was a shampoo I had bought on our trip to Abbeytown the previous day. I had put it in our car's back seat organiser. This morning Luca asked me what I had done with the shampoo. I had made a "mistake" again. I saw Luca making a face as if he was experiencing severe pain. He stiffened and clenched his fists. For him, the world was falling apart because I had brought "poison" into our house again.

Luca had "decontaminated" our whole car during his previous cleansing activities. However, he had overseen the car back seat organiser, where he had always put pens and other utensils on his way back from school. Therefore, the inside of the organiser was contaminated, and so was the shampoo bottle I had brought into our house. Although I had washed my hands after our shopping trip, Luca was worried that the kitchen, his food and his body could be contaminated. His fear was exasperating me. Once more, I was talking against a wall in my efforts to talk some sense into him.

I went for a walk with Rover to gain some distance. When I returned, Luca was still sitting in an armchair and was completely tensed up. I asked him what was underneath his worry. He thought about it how he could best explain it to me. Then he said it was actually quite simple: "When I was feeling so bad, even before the colitis, I always was afraid of being useless and that I would never be able to fulfil my plans. When it was going on for years that I never had enough energy, I was always told that I was only making it up. It is a fact that during this time, I often felt as if I would faint. Sometimes I could hardly climb stairs, but all the same, I dragged myself to football training.

I was afraid and alone with my fear because nobody took me seriously. Then, when the bloody diarrhoea appeared, I thought the chemicals from school had destroyed my body. I was afraid that maybe I had to die. I was glad when I received my colitis diagnosis because at least you don't die from this illness. And now that I am finally feeling better after all these years, I am afraid that the school poison will make me sick again. I want to become a football player. That's all I want." Once again, his face was turning into a painful grimace. His face and posture expressed what it looked like in the rest of his body and maybe in every individual cell. Finally, Luca began to cry, and I was glad about it. He hadn't cried in a long time, a far too long time. I cried with him.

11th of May:

The spell of fine weather is over. A thick layer of clouds has covered the blue sky. The clouds have swallowed the upper third of "our" mountain. No air movement; everything is still, besides the twittering of the birds. The hawthorn is flowering abundantly everywhere this spring. Its sea of blossoms is silhouetted against the grey-blue mountain. It is as if nature was wearing a romantic, lightly floating bridal veil.

The night before, I had the following dream: Luca and I were staying with my mother in

Germany. We walked into the town and crossed the main street. Luca was eating an apple. He kicked the apple core away with a "rabona shot" in a long curving arc. A boy of Luca's age came towards us. Amazed and excited, he said: "Have I just seen right? What a shot!" Another slightly older guy stretched out his hand to congratulate Luca. He asked him where he was playing football. Then he said: "We would need somebody like you in our team." Luca looked at him with big eyes and an astonished smile. I was standing there next to him, just feeling so happy.

Then I woke up. I looked at the alarm clock: 7:30 pm. I had to cry and could hardly calm myself down. Alex didn't know what was happening, and I couldn't explain it to him right away. Everything could be so simple, but we seemed stuck in a deadlock here in Ireland. Luca has had many bad experiences and has often been confronted with the resentment of others. He had constantly felt that he needed to justify himself for everything. Even his "best friend" had always been jealous, and Luca wasn't a show-off. In his new school, one of his jealous classmates kicked Luca aggressively when the boys were playing football while the others were watching. Only a few girls protested and stood up for Luca, who didn't defend himself. Afterwards, in the changing room, someone sprayed his deodorant on Luca. He was often called "gay" only because he behaved differently.

Situations in which Luca had been insulted and harassed and about which he had only told me months after their occurrence were now appearing in my imagination. I noticed how my empathy for Luca and my pain transformed into rage. I was angry that Luca had to become so ill and about his social environment's role in this. The bullying in the school had meant a massive attack on his integrity, and it was no surprise that his inner centre – his gut – had been entirely thrown out of balance.

And then I remembered what Mairead had explained about the law of attraction: pain bodies (bullying victims) attract other pain bodies (bullying perpetrators) because pain wants to be fed. Luca had been an easy victim as he was unwell and isolated. Perpetrators can feel this; they actually sense it. Mairead said that Luca had to learn to set his boundaries and not to play the victim role, as otherwise, other people would always dump their trash on him. She was convinced you can also get contaminated by emotional injuries and what others say and do to you. If you absorb this hurt without defending yourself and setting clear boundaries, you quasi-contaminate yourself. She believed that the "contaminated, poisoned school utensils" symbolised the hurt inflicted on Luca. When another pupil had poured chemicals, of all things, on Luca, it must have been like a nightmare for him. The law of attraction?

An essential function of the gastrointestinal tract's membrane is the establishment of a boundary between inside and outside and the body's protection from harmful environmental influences. This membrane is our largest contact surface with the environment. However, it only has one cell layer thickness, making it very vulnerable and potentially susceptible to foreign invaders. Therefore about 70 per cent of our immune system is located in the gut. The digestive tract is the front line at which the immune system comes into contact with bacteria, viruses and fungi. Here, our immune cells learn to distinguish between "self" and "non-self" and are trained to attack harmful invaders. At the same time, the immune system needs to have a finely adjusted tolerance towards the gut flora.

Is it possible that for Luca's body-mind-soul-system, the gut had become where he tried to protect himself against the negative energy and the toxic atmosphere he felt surrounded by? And in all its efforts to protect him, had his immune system overreacted, provided for never-ending inflammation, and given the red alert? Certainly, all these factors had played a role in Luca developing colitis of all diseases and not any other one. Also, the timing of his illness is very telling.

To be bullied means stress on a mental, emotional and physical level. Acute stress leads to a whole cascade of bodily changes known as the fight-or-flight response. This reaction is triggered to protect us. When the brain perceives a situation as threatening, it stimulates our adrenal glands to secrete cortisol. This stress hormone prepares us for fight or flight, and amongst other things, it causes our blood pressure to increase, our heart rate to accelerate, and our blood sugar levels to go up. At the same time, elevated cortisol levels impact the function of our immune system and the digestive tract.

Although the fight-or-flight reaction can be crucial for survival, it can also make us ill and even threaten our lives if it is permanently on and if a relaxation response is not taking place as an antidote. Stress is regarded as being involved in the development of almost any illness. It not only makes us more susceptible to disease but also hinders the body in its attempts to heal itself.

Permanent stress is associated with a wide range of health conditions, including autoimmune diseases. A danger of excessive cortisol production is that this stress hormone opens the mucosal membrane's tight junctions, leading to increased gut permeability. The leaky gut syndrome again throws the doors wide open for autoimmune diseases, including inflammatory bowel disease. *(4)* Added to this, emotional states like anger or fear and the resulting stress can promote the virulence of bacteria and viruses and enhance their reproduction. *(5)*

Once again, feelings of regret and grief came over me because Luca had been forced to return to Ireland and could not stay in Germany. It had been so good for him to feel accepted and more grounded. Over there, when he arrived at a football field, he was asked if he wanted to join in. Here in Ireland, he was greeted with a: "Who the fuck is this?"

Out of the blue, a pulsating pain ran through my knee without apparent reason. I could directly experience the link between emotional and physical pain. It saddened me deeply that everything had turned out the way it had. Luca's pain was my pain. How was I supposed to handle it?

Despite all my efforts to protect Luca as much as possible, I had to agree with the Danish family therapist and author Jesper Juul who said: "No matter how much we are trying to get everything right for our children, life is not always easy – also not for children. We can love our children and try to teach them as well as we can how to face life, but we cannot protect them from being. Suffering is part of every human life [...] *(6)*."

Diary-Entry of 12th May:
From a gut point of view, everything is well, but the contamination phobia was a considerable problem once again. I hope Luca gets a grip on his anxiety because I find it hard to handle the strain on my nerves. I am immensely frustrated

that I cannot help Luca with his phobia. Today I became angry, not so much because of Luca but of the whole situation. Out of pure frustration, I pedalled up the mountain on my bike in the rain, which had a very liberating effect on me. When I returned home, Luca had cut his hair really short, although he only got a professional haircut a few days ago. I asked him if this made him feel better. He said he would wear his hair close-cropped as long as he felt unhappy. He told me about his fear that one day he might, after all, have made it as a football player and might be playing in a higher league just to become ill again. I was shocked by the extent of his lack of confidence and his negative thinking.

Diary-Entry of 28th May:
Since his last flare-up (2 months ago), Luca has put on almost four kilograms. He is pleased about it, and so am I.

Letting Go

During the following weeks, Luca was under a lot of stress again because he felt he had to continue his cleaning jobs. For a short time, his football training had distracted him from this obsession. I let him do it, hoping it would help him somehow.

During another conversation about his contamination phobia, I explained to Luca that he had to show his body more confidence. I told him that he should treat his body like his best friend rather than give out to it when it showed any weakness. "You can only expect a good and fruitful relationship with your friends if you treat them with love, respect and confidence. In the same way, we have to see the relationship with our body and every single cell that makes it," I said to Luca and asked him how he would behave if someone criticised him all the time and did not think him capable of doing anything right. "You would feel hurt and withdraw from this person, wouldn't you?" I continued.

I explained to Luca that his body had a universal intelligence and extraordinary self-healing abilities, with the immune system and detoxification processes all part of this. I told him that he could trust these abilities and had to trust them. "Even if your body takes in any toxins, a healthy body is well able to get rid of them again. You must believe this; by doing so, you will strengthen these abilities rather than undermine them with your fear."

I tried to convince him that his fear was contra productive and that fear, in general, wasn't a good guide for his life. I had an idea and made the following suggestion to him: He should try to set his 17th birthday in the next month as a deadline. Until then, he had to be finished with his cleaning jobs. On the night before his birthday, at midnight, we would perform the following ritual: He should write all his fears on a sheet of paper and then burn it in the fire. That could help him to let go of his fear. I explained to him that he was not identical to his fear but that his fears were only his beliefs. Luca liked my proposal. He wanted to work at it.

During my next session with Mairead, we again discussed Luca's contamination phobia. She doubted that we could solve his anxiety problem on our own. She didn't believe that I was up to this task. My fruitless attempts would only frustrate me and rob me of the energy I needed for Luca and myself. She thought that Luca needed the support of a professional. I explained to her that Dr Morrin had referred Luca to a psychotherapist but that the waiting time for an appointment was very long. Mairead advised me to put pressure on Dr Morrin again. She said it was obvious that we were all suffering immensely from Luca's contamination phobia, which negatively impacted our family life.

I followed Mairead's advice and rang the psychologist to whom – at least according to Dr Morrin – Luca had been referred half a year ago. I was utterly perplexed when I was told that Luca's name wasn't even on the waiting list and that we had been waiting for the appointment in vain. It was very bizarre. When Luca would have needed a thorough physical examination by which one could have found out about his dysbiosis and possible food sensitivities, he had been referred to a psychologist and had been asked to take psychiatric drugs. At that point, the progression of his physical symptoms could have been stopped or even reversed. And now we didn't get an appointment, although he was facing a severe mental problem, and we desperately needed support.

7th of June 2017, Luca's 17th Birthday:

Today it is 17 years ago that Luca was born. After waking up, I thanked the universe for being blessed with this beautiful gift. I laid the breakfast table and decorated it with the flowers that Alex had bought. I placed a candle on the table and put Luca's presents and his birthday card beside it.

I remembered how bad he had felt on his last birthday, even though he didn't have full-blown colitis then. This year Luca was in good form and remarked: "If someone had told me last year that I would have so much energy on my 17th birthday and that I could make so much progress with my football training, but that the price would be having to go through hell for ten months, I would have said: Yes, okay, I am ready."

After lunch, Luca wanted to go down to the pitch. The weather was not bad, at least it wasn't raining. Another boy was taking shots at one goal. I noticed Luca was getting nervous and hesitant and that he might wonder if he still wanted to go to the pitch. I said: "Luca, it's the summer holiday, and it's likely that you will meet other kids here. You have big plans, don't you? You can't always turn back." He agreed with me.

We went along the football pitch as far as the place where Luca always climbed over the fence. The other boy raised his hand, and we returned his greeting. I asked Luca, "Why don't you exchange a few words with him? Behave as you would consider normal when you come to a pitch where others are training, too. Conduct yourself as you wished somebody else would behave towards you."

I walked on and climbed up a high dune. The calm ocean lay in front of me. In the diffuse light, all the colours appeared pale. I walked barefoot to the edge of the water. I closed my eyes and breathed in and out very consciously. I became one with the surrounding nature and the rhythmic breathing of the sea. I felt peaceful and at ease and was confident everything would be alright again. On the way back, I collected Luca. The other boy had gone. Luca told me they had talked briefly. "He was quite nice, actually. I think I know his older brother from school. He was one of the few ones who were okay. They are from Dublin."

A week after his birthday, Luca had an appointment with Dr Cody at the university clinic. We had to wait two hours in a dark, stuffy corridor until our turn. While Luca was creating a thumbnail for his new football video on his smartphone, I was reading a chapter in Bruce Lipton's "Biology of Belief". It was about conventional medicine's refusal to accept alternative methods like energy healing or homoeopathy.

At first, Lipton explained that drugs always have adverse effects as it is impossible to direct and restrict their action precisely. In comparison, hormones like histamine or oestrogen are produced in the body only where and for as long as needed. However, their artificially manufactured equivalents, which we take as drugs, reach the whole body. They also affect cells, tissues and organs that are not intended as their target. You cannot outperform nature's intelligence.

According to Lipton, in the USA alone, the side effects of prescription drugs are responsible for more than 300,000 deaths yearly. *(1)* He calls this a disturbing statistic for representatives of a healing profession who, at the same time, refuse to appreciate the potential of energy healing methods which are gentle and free from side effects. He accuses conventional Western medicine of being reductionist and arrogant. It ignored the findings of quantum physics and had a mechanistic, strictly materialistic concept of the human body, which left no space for the spirit and immaterial energy.

Although many scientists, through the latest technology, show that life is closely connected with invisible energy fields, the conventional medical world doesn't acknowledge that energy plays a crucial role in our bodily functions and health. Energy healing methods are not profitable for the pharmaceutical industry. Therefore their exploration is minimal, which makes it possible to marginalise them as "unscientific". (The same can be said about dietary healing approaches.)

Ironically, modern imaging diagnostics (for instance, magnetic resonance imaging or computer tomography) use precisely the fact that our tissues and organs send out a specific energy spectrum. Diseased tissue has another energy than healthy tissue, and this is how it can be identified.

Our body-mind-soul-system is permanently surrounded by an energy field and sends out energy. We react to energies, which can have a constructive (energy enhancing) or destructive (energy reducing) effect. The difference between good vibes and bad vibes is something that everyone knows from their own experience. It makes a big difference whether you are with like-minded people having a good time or in an environment that is depleting your energy.

The latter fittingly described the atmosphere that surrounded us. Once again, Luca hit the nail on the head when he said: "While you have to wait here in this dark hole for hours, you could even forget your name." When we were called up, we were just about able to remember it.

After what had felt like an eternity, we finally sat vis-a-vis Dr Cody. We informed him that Luca had discontinued his medications over two months ago due to many severe adverse effects. I started to list them but was very soon interrupted by Dr Cody, who wanted to know how Luca was at present. Luca answered that he was well and emphasised that he was still on his diet. Dr Cody passed the brief comment that in some patients, dietary interventions show positive results. That was all.

He filled out a form that Luca needed for the ensuing blood sampling. I asked him if Luca's cholesterol level could also be tested. I intended to explain the reason for this as – according to the GAPS diet – Luca was eating a lot of eggs. But our time was already up. Dr Cody told us that Luca would get another routine appointment in a year, and just like that, we were out of the door again.

We had been waiting two hours for this conversation, which only lasted about five minutes. I had been naïve enough to believe Dr Cody would be interested in Luca's experience. Luca was symptom-free without taking any medications (or maybe this was the reason why). The diet with which he had achieved his remission had been scientifically studied. However, this medical specialist didn't show the slightest interest in hearing about it. I had expected that it would be Dr Cody's highest aim to support the recovery of his patients through interventions that are as natural as possible and do no harm. That is especially desirable for young patients such as Luca.

I found it very sad that Dr Cody was not more curious and eager to learn from his patients, as this makes any therapist move forward and determines their quality in the end. I was also shocked by his lack of empathy. I was perplexed and felt enormously disappointed. At the same time, however, I was infinitely grateful that we were following our path and were not dependent on conventional medicine. If physicians were listening properly to what their patients had to say and gathering and analysing their valuable observations, mainstream medicine could have advanced further in chronic inflammatory bowel disease. What we had experienced during our medical appointment reinforced my notion that the conventional medical system has no sincere interest in supporting patients in reversing their condition. It is only designed to manage the rising number of sick people and to treat their symptoms.

We walked through the town to the parking

lot. It was overcast and rainy. The cold wind was blowing in our faces, and it felt like autumn, although it was only mid-June. We had just reached the car when the rain started pouring down. We were in a hurry because the shops would soon be closing and we wanted to buy a football as a small treat for Luca.

On our drive home, Luca asked if I had noticed the young fellow sitting opposite him in the waiting area. I said I had only perceived him marginally. He was more lying in his seat than sitting. On his arrival, he first got himself a large coffee. He wasn't looking well at all and seemingly was in pain. Luca had overheard a phone call between the guy and supposedly one of his mates. "Do you know what he said, Mama?" – "No, tell me," I replied, and Luca began: "I had these feckin' symptoms again. Had to take them old steroids. Took a few days until they kicked in. Shall we go for a few pints and have some craic?" – "What?" I said. "Beer during a flare-up? And alcohol while being on steroids?"

Luca was also shocked and noted that this was probably how most patients dealt with their illnesses. He assumed that many patients would rather throw in pills than take responsibility for their health by making meaningful lifestyle changes. I replied that this was also because important information was being withheld from them, and they were being intimidated. "That guy was probably only 22 years old and looked completely knackered. Luckily we have a different approach. I am so glad you are helping me become well again," said Luca.

In the evening, I was preoccupied with digesting our visit to the doctor. I felt utterly exhausted. The few hours in the hospital had sapped the energy out of me, and I asked myself how a sick person was supposed to recover from an illness in such a dark and stuffy atmosphere. Having to stay in the hospital would be an absolute nightmare for me. I went to bed early and slept like a baby.

Already on the following day, Dr Cody's assistant rang to tell me the results of the blood test. At least this service left nothing to be desired. Luca's blood, cholesterol and liver values were all normal. His inflammation markers were down. One of his kidney values was slightly elevated, but according to the nurse, this was nothing to worry about. However, we should watch this value on the occasion of the next blood test.

I felt relieved and went for a walk on our property, a short sunny intermezzo with a warm breeze. Unintentionally, I startled two wild doves and could hear their wings flapping when they fluttered away. The vibrant pink of the foxgloves, which had opened their blossoms. The twittering of birds from the hedgerow. The mooing of a cow in the distance. The yellow lilies and buttercups swaying softly in the wind. The sound of rustling leaves. The murmur of our stream. I soaked up everything. I was happy and felt confirmed that we were doing the right thing. A feeling of boundless gratitude was flowing through me.

Luca had finished his cleaning jobs in the house, or at least, this is what he said. He had worked through the seemingly endless list of objects in his head which were definitely or possibly contaminated. He no longer felt pressured to control every move Alex or I made in the kitchen, and he didn't have to clean before I prepared his meals.

That was a great relief for me and made everything a lot easier. Nevertheless, I knew that he was still very vulnerable and that it only needed a small trigger to destabilise the peace. I also was apprehensive that Luca's fear would focus on something new now, namely his bladder or kidneys. I was annoyed with myself for mentioning the elevated kidney value in his presence and thus arousing his concern.

28th of June, visit to Dr Morrin:

Since his appointment with Dr Cody, Luca had suffered from painful urination and constant hot feet. Therefore I proposed that we hand in a urine sample at Dr Morrin's clinic to ensure he didn't have a bladder infection. That was the best method to tame Luca's fear. A few days afterwards, I went to Dr Morrin to talk to him about Luca's elevated kidney value and the result of his urine test.

Dr Morrin told me that the urine test had shown no abnormalities. He said there was no need to worry about the elevated kidney value and that it had nothing to do with increased urinary frequency or painful urination. However, this didn't explain where Luca's symptoms originated from. (A few days later, they had disappeared on their own.)

I also mentioned the obscurities concerning Luca's referral to the psychotherapist. I asked Dr Morrin to refer him again. I talked with Dr Morrin about Luca's contamination phobia and the relationship I saw between his anxiety and his colitis. I said we had to get a grip on his contamination phobia; otherwise, his gut wouldn't heal either.

Dr Morrin's only comment was that I shouldn't over-interpret everything. Once again, I was speechless. I know Luca better than anybody else does. I have observed him every day since he came into my life. We have a very deep relationship, and often we find out that we had just been thinking the same thing. I am always trying to understand what is going on inside Luca mentally, spiritually, and physically and how these factors interact. I wasn't in the least over-interpreting anything!

I was annoyed with Dr Morrin. Did he think he could help his patients with his pigeonhole thinking and reductionist approach, which didn't acknowledge that everything is deeply connected? After I had gained some distance again, I felt it was a terrible pity that he was so stuck in his conventional medicine thought prison.

Ironically, just before my conversation with Dr Morrin, I had read a chapter in Bruce Lipton's "Biology of Belief" about the power of the mind. The impact of positive beliefs on the body is scientifically proven in every pharmaceutical trial when there is a verifiable improvement of a patient's symptoms after the treatment with a placebo (a fake medication). The effect of a positive attitude and positive expectations on the healing process could also be proven using fake operations. According to Bruce Lipton, at least 30 per cent of all humans are susceptible to the "placebo effect", as it is called. *(2)*

This phenomenon has always been a thorn in the side of the pharmaceutical industry because, in a placebo-controlled study, the effect of the "real" drug has to be superior to that of the placebo. And this is the only way to prove its efficacy. However, only 20 per cent of conventional drugs are supposed to be more efficient than placebos. *(3)*

Already Jesus is supposed to have said that what we experience depends on what we believe (Mt 9, 29 "According to your faith be it unto you."). If our conviction that we can be healed is strong enough, it can happen. Conversely, we can think ourselves into being ill. Initially, I only had a vague suspicion that there must be a link between Luca's thoughts and emotions and his colitis. In the meantime, however, I did not doubt that Luca's fears and negative thinking were manifesting in his gut.

As long as he was terrified because he was deeply convinced that he was poisoning himself, it was no surprise that his immune system was also on red alert and entirely off track. As mentioned before, toxins in our digestive tract can cause gut inflammation and bloody diarrhoea. Maybe Luca's digestive system didn't distinguish between real and "imagined" poison. Maybe his gut was reacting to the feeling of a massive threat, no matter if this was real or just imaginary.

What has been acknowledged in Eastern medicine for over 5 000 years and has therefore influenced its medical treatment methods can be verified in numerous scientific studies today: the body and the mind are inextricably linked. Consequently, it would be adequate to speak of the "body-mind-system" or the "body-mind-soul-system". However, Western orthodox medicine still regards the body and the mind as separate entities. The body is seen as similar to a machine that can be detached into its various parts. These parts can be repaired or treated by an ever-growing amount of different specialists. For physical conditions, we have physicians, and for emotional or mental problems, we have psychologists.

19th of June, my last visit to Mairead:
I told her that Luca and I would return to Germany for an extended time. This decision was not something I had arrived at after long contemplation, but it had turned up spontaneously. Why had this option not come into my mind earlier? Probably because I had been so attached to the past and because my whole thinking had been going around in circles. Now I could let go of my self-accusations and emotional injuries and focus on the future again. I told Mairead that I had written my own prescription for Luca, and she asked me what it comprised. I tried to explain it to her. As it was Mairead who had drawn my attention to Dr Bruce Lipton, I began with the insights I had gained through him:

When we are tense, fearful, worried and stressed, our organism goes into "protection mode" right down to the cellular level. That is Bruce Lipton's conviction gained from decades-long research in cell biology focusing on human stem cells. The protection mode impairs growth and regeneration processes and inhibits the creation of life-sustaining energy, which can only happen in its opposite, the "growth mode".

Both fundamental survival mechanisms have developed over billions of years. What began in single-celled organisms is also essential for the survival of complex multicellular organisms like humans. Both mechanisms or responses are mutually exclusive. In the protection mode ("fight-or-flight"), it makes little sense to keep up processes of growth or regeneration. Also, the function of the immune system is compromised. The protection mode uses a lot of energy but does not produce any. Some processes only run minimally, such as the regeneration of intestinal cells. Under normal conditions, they are completely renewed after every 72 hours. However, in the protection mode, this process is restricted. The longer we are in this mode, the more our energy reserves get depleted, which can compromise our growth.

If we live in protection mode long-term, we significantly compromise our joy in living and our overall health. Lipton says that although it is possible to survive under stress, chronic inhibition of growth mechanisms has a massive impact on our vitality. And if we want to thrive, it is not enough to eliminate stressful factors from our lives. We must actively try to live a joyful and fulfilled life inspired by love. And this stimulates our growth response. Lipton is convinced that our beliefs, inner attitudes, and lifestyles impact the optimal functioning of our cells more significantly than our genetic make-up does. He says learning how to use our minds for growth is life's big secret. *(4)*

Reading Lipton's book made me aware that

Luca had lived in protection mode for years. We had to do everything possible to convert his organism into growth mode. Luca's diet is a crucial factor for becoming intact, whole and healthy again, but it is by far not the only one. Besides re-establishing his intestinal health, we want to improve his quality of life, vitality and inner peace.

I believe that the environment that made Luca ill cannot support him in becoming well again. We have to create a spatial distance to his "toxic" environment. If his extreme fear and the stress reactions caused by it keep catching up with him, his gut won't be able to heal. As long as he keeps thinking and feeling the same things, his brain's corresponding patterns and circuits will strengthen, making it increasingly difficult to break them. I hope he can replace his automated and self-sabotaging thinking patterns with new and positive experiences. Our experiences shape our brains, and their plasticity is highest at a young age.

However, Luca must solve the problems created by his emotional, thinking and behavioural patterns on a deeper level of consciousness. He won't be able to escape from unpleasant situations or feelings for all his life, especially not from himself. We are constantly bringing ourselves to every place our life takes us. I will encourage Luca to discover what hinders him from living in tune with his true self.

Luca is fully committed to becoming a

football player and shall have his chance. I will do everything to support him on his way. He shall at least be able to try out what is possible for him. I want to create the conditions that help him achieve his goals and give him the feeling that he has more control over his life. I believe that feelings of helplessness and powerlessness have gained predominance in the past years and have promoted the development of his anxiety. Compulsive cleaning is an attempt to gain a sense of control and safety. He may no longer need his compulsive behaviour if things go well for him, giving him a feeling of stability. Over time, he will also learn that many things in life are beyond our control. Instead of obsessively creating an illusion of safety, he will learn to entrust himself to life's flow and rely on his inner resources. He will replace fear with hope and optimism.

I am deeply convinced that there is a very close connection between self-fulfilment and health. I also believe that Luca's illness is closely related to his inability to express and fulfil himself. To make matters worse, he blamed himself for it. Seen from the outside, he had a happy childhood and was very much loved by us, but inside, he experienced disharmony and inner conflict. He was too young to articulate and discuss his problems with us. We will make good for this now, and I will take much time to listen to him. The word "guilt" or "guilty" is something we won't use any more. We all try to give our best whenever we can. We may not blame and punish ourselves if things are not going as planned. Getting up again after a setback and learning from our mistakes are the only things we can do.

It makes Luca happy if he can train in football and can make progress. He loves to get into a state of "flow" and to get completely lost in this feeling. We will use this sense of flow therapeutically for him. In a state of flow, you feel ecstatic, which by its very nature, excludes feelings of depression or anxiety. Being in this state invites feelings of serenity and deep relaxation while being highly concentrated at the same time. Being in a state of flow is similar to meditating. It is a wonderful medicine for Luca, and he shall be able to experience it as much as possible to heal himself.

I will also encourage him to be more creative. As a child, he loved to draw and paint. It was a balm for my soul when he was wholly absorbed in his creative process and humming happily, oblivious to everything around him.

Luca shall practise self-care and do the things which give him a feeling of physical and emotional well-being. I will have his back until he is perfectly healthy again. I will let him feel my unconditional love and let him be. He will attempt to protect himself from destructive influences and will work on setting his boundaries. He will only engage with people who relate to him with love, empathy and solidarity. We will keep any pressure from the outside away and create a cocoon-like protected space for him. Not forever, but as long as he needs it for healing himself and as long as it is doing him good. I hope that one day, an extraordinary butterfly will emerge from the cocoon.

Luca will also try to work on his personal development. He will learn to practise mindfulness and to live in the present moment, aware and without judgement. He will learn to observe his thoughts and feelings and to deal with them consciously. We will practise relaxation methods together because I have to become much more serene, too. I want to invite more fun, joy and laughter into our lives and embed practising gratitude firmly into our daily routine.

I will encourage Luca to write his own prescription for himself. What does he need to get healthy? What would be necessary that he could live an authentic life in tune with his "inner pilot light"? (This expression does not originate from me but from the American physician Lissa Rankin, author of "Mind over Medicine".) Which beliefs and behaviour patterns are blocking his way of getting there? Does he love and accept himself? Who would he be without his fears and self-criticism? Without his fear of not being good enough or of being disliked and excluded? Without the feeling of always having to justify himself and explain why he does certain things in a certain way? What would it be like if he could be himself and love himself in his uniqueness? How would it feel if he could trust the flow of life a bit more?

I will book two flights to Germany – one way! We will leave everything open and see how things go. Alex will keep everything running in Ireland and support us from there.

Mairead was very impressed. We also discussed my plans to write a book. She thought it was a great idea and that it was necessary to tell other people about our experiences and encourage them to take their health into their own hands and take responsibility for themselves and their lives. I told her I had already started working on it. With a smile, I added I would handle it like the bestselling author and great teacher of the West, Dr Wayne Dyer. I said I had already designed the book cover with the title and that I could see the finished book in my mind's eye. Now all that was left to do was to write it.

Mairead laughed. She asked me if there was anything else she could do for me. I told her I felt I could master my path on my own again. She said I could ring her anytime if I needed her support. Then she wished the three of us all the best. When we said goodbye, we hugged each other. "Thank you, Mairead, thank you for everything," I said to her and wished her well from the bottom of my heart. Only much later did I realise how meaningful our conversations had been for me. They saved me from becoming ill myself.

29th of June:

Luca and I were in Abbeytown together. Luca wanted to get a haircut. It was a good sign that he was interested in his appearance again. I remembered how he had shaved his head after his last visit to the barber. When Luca was ready at the hairdresser, we could get hold of some cool sportswear on sale. Luca was happy, and so was I. We had not been shopping together in ages because he hadn't been well enough. On this night, it got late. I was sitting in front of the fire listening to music. It was exactly one year since we went to Germany for our summer holidays. Looking back, it had been a year in which we all learned a lot.

Before bed, I went to the bathroom to get ready. I watched the clear night sky through the roof window. I saw a bright point and observed its slow motion. It must have been a satellite. Suddenly, a shooting star flashed by. I smiled and made a wish.

Toad Dream

Luca's final flare-up was in October 2017, not long until our departure to Germany. The last time that he had suffered from bloody diarrhoea was half a year ago. In the meantime, he had put on ten kilograms and had trained three to four hours daily. Luca looked healthy and athletic. His weight was perfect, and he had gained a lot of muscle. As he was physically well, his contamination phobia had also calmed down. However, it could come up again. Luca still had received no support from a psychotherapist.

The first signs of his forthcoming flare-up were a gurgling in the abdomen, flatulence and thinner stools than usual. I told Luca that this wasn't something to worry about yet. However, the next morning, he came into our bedroom and woke us up with the following words: "I wished I didn't have to say so, but I have bloody diarrhoea again." I took it with composure, and so did Luca. "I am glad to know where I stand now. I found it much harder to bear the feeling of uncertainty during the previous days," he continued. "I will get up shortly," I said. "Give me a few minutes. I'll be there for you in a moment."

I needed more time to be completely present. I took a few slow and conscious breaths. I still needed to process Luca's information fully. He was hungry and wanted to eat a bowl of soup. Fortunately, I had prepared a large pot of chicken soup the previous evening. Since his last flare-up in March, Luca had wanted no chicken soup. He had had enough of it, and it reminded him of his illness. I had accepted it, although the soup would have been good for him.

The previous weekend, I had cooked the "magic chicken soup" for our beloved dog Rover, who suffered from arthritis and could hardly walk. He also refused to eat his usual food, and I wanted to help him. I was worried about the old chap and feared we might have to euthanise him. Losing him would have been the last thing I had wished for before our departure to Germany. However, his self-healing abilities were astonishing. After three days of chicken soup with oat flakes and egg yolks, a few doses of arnica globuli, and a lot of tender loving care, he could go for a short walk with me again. His condition improved day by day. That is how we had re-discovered the well-tried chicken soup and why I had some ready for Luca. I hadn't expected it would serve him as a remedy for another flare-up. Now I was glad that I could offer it to him.

We returned to phase 1 of the GAPS diet. We knew what to expect and what to do. The first day of the flare-up was relatively mild. Luca had three bowel movements per day. In the night, his symptoms got very severe. Luca wanted to sleep in the living room on the couch. It allowed him to find a position with less pain than on his bed. He asked me if I could stay with him. I didn't mind and slept in a recliner. Luca had to go to the toilet every two to three hours. He had diarrhoea, which contained a lot of bloody mucus. On the following day, we stopped counting his bowel movements. Luca kept walking around that day because he had hardly any pain in an upright position. Altogether, this flare-up had not been as painful as the previous ones. I contacted our homoeopath again and asked him to send us the lycopodium globuli. Only the thought that there was help for him on the way helped Luca relax. His diet comprised chicken soup with carrots, turmeric, freshly ground black pepper and Himalayan salt, which contains many valuable trace minerals. He was drinking ginger, peppermint and chamomile tea alternately.

The following night, Luca's gut had calmed down again. He had only two bowel movements and could compensate for the lost sleep. On the third day of his flare-up, Luca felt significantly better. For breakfast, he had scrambled eggs. During the day, Luca ate chicken soup, and in the evening, he had chicken breast with mashed carrots and pumpkin. He only had three bowel movements during the day and could sleep the whole night.

On the following day, we continued with the same foods. Luca also started taking the homoeopathic remedy again. As far as his gut was concerned, this day went exceptionally well. However, his contamination phobia was so extreme that he couldn't find any rest with all his cleaning. That was not only exhausting for him but also challenging for Alex and me. I tried to pull myself together. I didn't want another argument because Luca needed peace for his gut to heal. His fear pulled me down a lot. I wished so much I had never told him about the leaky gut syndrome! Now he was anxious again that "the poison" (the school chemicals) could enter his bloodstream.

After four days, Luca's flare-up was over, and his stool returned to normal. We were sure this flare-up had been so mild because Luca's gut mucosa had healed and was much healthier. If the intestinal cells are optimally nourished and cared for, they regenerate every three days.

We compared the recent flare-up to the last one in March when Luca was still on his prescribed medication. Before, the flare-ups had occurred every two to three weeks. Since Luca had gone off his medication, he had been in remission for half a year. Another difference was that his recent flare-up lasted only four days and was relatively mild. Only on two of the four days had it been more severe. In comparison, Luca's flare-up in March had dragged on for two weeks and had immediately improved after discontinuing his medication.

That is not intended to encourage patients

to follow our example and discontinue their medications as rigorously as we had done it. And as mentioned before, this step should be discussed with a physician. I am also not claiming that our path is the only one that is right. Every disease course is different, and every patient has different needs. In Luca's case, however, his chances of gaining back his health were much better without the prescribed medications and following a dietary approach. That is contrary to the conventional treatment method.

Luca and I assumed that another die-off reaction must have occurred in his gut. We visualised some mutinous rebels still present in his intestines. Some of them had been forced to give up their position, but this was not happening without their resistance and release of dangerous toxins. I suspected that the trigger for this reaction was Luca's inner restlessness so shortly before our departure for Germany.

I also discovered that "opportunistic bacteria" could switch from a symbiotic or cooperative relationship to an aggressive one under stress. When their host is stressed, this doesn't leave the microbes unaffected, and they flip the lever. The fewer bacteria you have which are prone to a change of characteristics, the smaller the risk of a mutiny in the microbiome. Therefore, providing an excellent homestead to friendly gut bacteria is vital, as they act as a counterpart to opportunistic microbes. And this can be accomplished by having the right diet and consuming probiotic bacteria. *(1)*

I was relieved we had dealt with this flare-up relatively relaxed and confidently. I took Rover for a walk on our land. Autumn had arrived. My way led me through the rose arch into the small wood behind it, which had put on its autumnal robe and displayed a wide variety of colours. I picked up some particularly beautiful leaves and took them with me. I crossed the stream and, walking over the adjoining field, remembered a dream from a few months ago, which I had told Mairead at the time. It was set at the exact spot where I just had been. In my dream, a huge, ugly toad was sitting on the ground, which scared and disgusted me. I was almost petrified and didn't know what to do. Then a big bird came hovering along, and I wished it would snatch the toad and take it away. Then I woke up.

Mairead asked me how I would interpret this dream. I told her that the wild part of our land, which started behind the rose arch, was like a retreat for me. It was my "secret garden" where I observed nature, could forget the time and gain some distance. It was where I could take a deep breath, try to be in the present moment, get in touch with my inner core, and get new energy. The ugly toad, which you would find on a damp meadow beside a stream, symbolised Luca's illness, which had thrown me completely off track and severely threatened my inner peace. In my dream, I felt helpless and hoped to be rescued from the outside.

After listening to my explanations, Mairead asked me how it would be if I befriended the toad. At the time, her proposal didn't resonate with me, but now, on my walk, I suddenly realised that this was exactly what I had been doing for the past months. I wasn't the helpless victim any more who was yearning for salvation. Instead of resisting it, I had accepted Luca's illness as a challenge we could constantly learn from. This development has shown me how much wisdom there is in the Buddhist insight: suffering = pain x resistance. It is valid for mental and physical pain, likewise. Luca's illness had become a source of personal growth and inner wealth. After my walk, I placed the beautiful autumn leaves on the dining table. Luca admired them, and it made me happy to see that he appreciated their beauty.

Since Luca's flare-up in March, I had continued to extend my knowledge about ulcerative colitis. Never before has it been so easy to obtain valuable information as today. Often it is only a few mouse clicks away, and above all, for free. Of course, one should always check if a source is trustworthy. I had watched a few American video conferences online, such as "The Autoimmune Summit", "The Gluten Summit", and Dr Joseph Mercola's documentary series "Diet against Disease". The information I received from these sources validated we were following the right strategy for Luca. I came across some extremely competent Functional Medicine practitioners who generously make their knowledge available online. These included Chris Kresser, Dr Amy Myers, Dr Tom O'Bryan, Dr David Perlmutter, Dr Mark Hyman, Dr Michael T. Murray, Dr Zach Bush and Dr Michael Bush.

I also became aware that Luca's healing was a process that could take a very long time. Bringing 100 billion gut microbes back into equilibrium cannot be achieved quickly. A disease process, presumably going on for many years, might need as long to be reversed. Luca's illness didn't frighten us anymore because we could better understand its causes. We had learnt what we had overlooked before and what we could improve. Many autoimmune conditions can be reversed by diet and lifestyle changes.

I also looked into mindfulness and developed my personality further. When there is an obstacle in my way now, and I feel challenged, I try to gain some distance by taking a few conscious breaths. That helps me to relax and to be more in the present moment. It also improves blood flow in specific brain areas needed for a conscious reaction. In any situation, I try to maintain my focus on the following values, which should be the basis of every action: kindness, optimism, a constructive approach and forgiveness (towards yourself and others). Also, when faced with an unwelcome situation, my new approach is to ask myself what I can learn through it.

I observed that in the momentary situation in which Luca's new flare-up challenged me, I was much better equipped to stay calm and balanced. We had also become far more grateful. Instead of seeing Luca's latest flare-up as an unfairness of life and us as victims, we were grateful that Luca's gut had become far more robust again and could deal with the situation. And even if another flare should turn up in the future, we know how to tackle it and help Luca. It is a good feeling – one of safety and independence.

13th of October 2017:

Luca has overcome his flare-up, but his contamination phobia was extreme again, driving Alex and me nuts. For an external observer, it is almost impossible to imagine how this mental problem can paralyse a whole family. Once again, I had to escape, jumped on my bike and cycled along the solitary road below the mountain range that rises behind our property. Here it was wild and deserted. It was good for me to exercise and be out in nature: sheep, looking up and staring at me or just continuing to graze peacefully without taking any notice of me. The colour scheme, characterised by the warm hues of autumn leaves and the rusty roofs of abandoned cottages.

Usually, on these short trips, I could recharge my batteries, gain some distance and come back with new energy. This time, however, it wasn't the case. I felt like being stuck at a dead end. At home again, I lay down on my bed. I felt empty and heavy, and on this evening, I could have just stayed there. Since the start of Luca's illness, I had never felt like this. On this day, he emitted so much negative energy that I couldn't escape it either. His anxiety had him entirely under control. Not even the most profound arguments in the world could have helped to reduce it.

It was awkward. Luca's fear that "the poison" could make him ill sometime in the future made him ill right now. Once again, Luca's colitis appeared to me as a self-fulfilling prophecy. His disturbed intestinal flora, which we needed to restore, was only *one* aspect of his disease. As much as we can support our self-healing abilities and health with our positive thinking, we can also think ourselves into being ill or even dying. It frustrated me that even though I could help Luca on the physical level of his illness, I couldn't do it on the mental side of it.

Luca entered the room and sat down next to me on my bed. He was in despair. His fear was like a demon he couldn't escape from. He told me a few days before the beginning of his recent flare-up, he had been terrified of becoming ill again and not being able to go to Germany. He said he had truly felt how this fear was triggering something in his gut. Luca said: "It was like having a phone line between my brain and my belly and as if someone had rung down there to put everything in a state of turmoil." He had noticed how it had gurgled in his gut. Then flatulence and pain developed, and at some stage, the diarrhoea returned.

There was an interplay between Luca's fears, the stress reaction caused by this, and his colitis symptoms. And this corresponds to what the majority of IBD patients find. Most of them are convinced that psychological stress triggered their disease and was also responsible for their flare-ups. Particularly patients who are also suffering from anxiety and depression describe this relationship. *(2)*

We started talking about Luca's anxiety. He said that he always had a lot of fear. As a young child, he had been afraid of the darkness, later of burglars and then of diseases. He also told me how unhappy and lonely he had often been. In the company of other children, he had never really experienced a sense of belonging. He had often felt inadequate and inferior because he was not like them. When they devalued his clothes or utensils, which we had often bought during our holidays in Germany, it was the judgement of his classmates that counted. Their negative comments could refer to banal things such as pencils, erasers or sharpeners. Luca had always felt that he had to justify himself for everything. The thought that the others were simply jealous would never have occurred to him.

He told me he had always tried to perform at his best to receive recognition and acceptance. He had always wanted to be the best, be it in exams, in arts or sports. Of course, by having this attitude, he had put himself under enormous pressure and had created a very stressful life for himself. He said that he had never really felt that he belonged to Ireland. He had been tremendously bored at the weekends and in the endless summer holidays, especially if it had been raining for days on end. Then his loneliness, boredom, frustration and sadness got so unbearable that he sometimes provoked me. He knew which buttons to push and enjoyed it when I got angry and when he could ruin my day.

I knew Luca had no influence on his anxiety and that his present behaviour wasn't intended to annoy me. Anyhow, I probably reacted so sensitively and irritably to his compulsive disorder because it reminded me of these episodes from his childhood. Sometimes it felt like I had to deal with a naughty, stubborn child who did his best to be a real pain in the neck. I had to learn to let go of the past, also concerning this matter, and not let it impact what I was feeling in the present.

It was good to talk with Luca about his childhood experiences. As a child, he could not reflect on everything that made him unhappy. I took Luca in my arms and said to him: "Luca, you know I absolutely love you. I always have, and I always will. But the most important thing is that you love yourself because you are unique. Have the courage to be yourself. Be true to yourself, and don't worry about what other people say or think. Try to let go of the past and live as well as you can in the present moment."

On this evening, Luca took over the kitchen. He chopped and cooked his vegetables and baked his salmon. Then he ate the meal that he had prepared by himself with delight. Alex and I only had a bit of cheese and a glass of wine. I went to bed early. My conversation with Luca was still going through my head, and I wondered why fear dominated his life so much.

Maybe I had been overprotective and thus had given him the feeling that the world wasn't safe for him. Now he was seventeen and trying to take care of himself as well as possible. He was doing this with the precision characteristic of him and was going to extremes.

I believe Luca has already come into this world with much fear. I recall all those ultrasound scans during my pregnancy. Somehow, it made me nervous to hear Luca's heartbeat with the help of the technical gadgets. At the beginning of an ultrasound scan, I was still relatively relaxed, but in the course of it, Luca's heartbeat became faster and faster. The more nervous I got, the quicker his little heart raced. Sometimes it got so fast that I was afraid that it would burst. It never crossed my mind that my stress hormones were responsible for this.

Luca was born entirely healthy. During his first two weeks, he rested and slept most of the time. I was pleasantly surprised at how easy it was to live with a newborn. However, the peace was over from one day to the next when Luca got three-month baby colic. It must be a profound and distressing experience for such a tiny human being to be tormented by painful cramps daily. With the onset of the three-month colic, Luca stopped sleeping during the daytime.

It took him *eleven* and a half years to sleep through the night. Luca always had a very sharp mind, and surely his lack of basic trust was on the other side of the coin. When Luca was a toddler, an Irish nurse noted that he was a very alert child. Besides being bright, this also means that you are in a state of alert and on guard. So that was a very accurate description of Luca's disposition.

Jerome Kagan, a well-known American developmental psychologist, categorised the temperaments we are born with roughly into four archetypes: shy, bold, optimistic and melancholic. These temperaments mould the prevailing mood that is typical for our emotional life. They are based on a characteristic pattern of cerebral (referring to the brain or cerebrum) activity, but they are by no means our fate. According to Kagan, every fifth child has a shy or fearful temperament. *(3)*

Interestingly, he also observed in domestic cats that every seventh one is unusually timid and behaves similarly fearfully as shy children. Instead of being curious, these cats shy away from the unknown and only dare to approach small rodents. Scientists discovered that parts of the amygdala – an area of the brain where fear and anxiety are generated – are exceptionally excitable in these cats.

It is characteristic of shy kids that they are affected by paralysing fear in social situations, be it in kindergarten, in school or on the playground. They are uncommunicative and silently watch other children play. According to Kagan, these shy children often have other intense fears. They fear, for instance, that their house could burn down; they fear jumping into the swimming pool or being alone in the dark. They are also more prone to having nightmares.

These sensitive children are at a high risk of developing anxiety disorders as teenagers. They are terrified of new situations and get panic symptoms such as palpitations, difficulty breathing, fear of suffocation or the feeling that something terrible could happen to them or that they will die.

The nervous system of shy children is set to a far lower threshold level for the excitability of the amygdala than that of bold children. That is linked to the neurochemistry in their body. Kagan assumes that shy children have inherited a chronically high concentration of noradrenaline or other brain substances that activate the amygdala and thus level down its excitability threshold.

Kagan also found evidence that the sympathetic nervous system of shy children has a higher responsiveness than that of other children. This part of the autonomic nervous system primes the body for stressful or emergency situations (fight or flight). This higher responsiveness is reflected, for example, by higher blood pressure at rest or more significant dilation of the pupils up to an increased noradrenaline level in the urine. *(4)*

In his fascinating international bestseller "Emotional Intelligence", psychologist Daniel Goleman writes shy individuals seem to be born with a neuronal wiring that makes them react stronger even to mild stressors. From birth, their heart beats faster in reaction to a strange or new situation than that of other children. "This easily aroused anxiety seems to underlie their lifelong timidity: they treat any new person or situation as though it were a potential threat *(5)*," says Goleman.

It is probable that individuals who were timid as children are more predisposed to fear, worry and guilt when middle-aged than their extroverted contemporaries. Also, stress-related health problems such as migraines, irritable stomach or other stomach complaints are more likely. However, according to Kagan, no one is condemned to remain the same way as they were born. It is possible to correct the over-anxiousness one was born with and tame the amygdala through positive life experiences. That is thanks to our brain's high plasticity, which allows its neural networks to change through growth and reorganisation for as long as we live.

I am convinced that Luca's colitis had much to do with his lack of (basic) trust and grounding. Even today, he prefers to be in an environment that is familiar to him. That also allows him to unlock his full potential. New situations have always made him anxious. In general, he preferred to be among adults rather than children, as the latter were more unpredictable. During his entire childhood, Luca had tried to put down roots or find a good "fit". At some times, this was easier for him than at others. Although he brought valuable personality traits into relationships, he never received the due appreciation from his so-called "friends". That is sad because positive experiences with peers are precisely what help a shy and timid child to feel accepted and to become more self-confident.

I had often compared Luca with a plant which cannot flourish and prosper to the same extent in any environment. Sometimes I saw him as a rose which is very adorable but thorny as well. Scientists have also drawn a comparison between children and flowers. According to studies, some children profit more from a friendly, empathetic environment than others. However, they also suffer more from negative experiences. Scientists reminded this of flowers, and they classified children roughly into what they called "dandelion children" and "orchid children".

Dandelion children are robust. They can put down roots everywhere and can also thrive under bad conditions. Orchid children, on the other hand, are very sensitive, as the comparison implies. If poorly treated, they can't develop as well and can have lifelong problems. "In a greenhouse, however, under good conditions, they blossom wonderfully. If orchid children grow up without stress, they can develop even better than their more robust peers, who remain less receptive to external influences, including positive ones *(6)*," explains the psychotherapist and author Sabine Wery von Limont.

Without any doubt, Luca was an orchid child. At home with us, he always had greenhouse conditions. However, he also had to learn to thrive outside this protected environment. That had always been a big challenge for him and had been associated with a lot of inner tension and stress. These "emotional residuals" from his childhood were undoubtedly involved in developing his illness, which had not occurred overnight.

On the following morning, Luca woke us

up. He had already been cleaning for an hour to make the kitchen and the rest of our house safe for him again. He was in a much better mood, and we passed the day peacefully. Luca helped me in the kitchen to have me better under his control. Luckily, my nerves were strong enough to simply go along with it. There were only twelve days left until our departure to Germany. I was optimistic again that we could make it there. We had a lot of preparations to make. We couldn't waste any of our energy and had to act in a positive and constructive manner.

During the days prior to our departure, it got very stressful again because Luca didn't want us to take anything "contaminated" with us to Germany. He cleaned everything before it was put in the suitcase, and then it had to remain there. I had my doubts that his gut could bear all that stress. Even the night before our departure, I was unsure if we could travel the following day.

My equanimity surprised me. I was ready to see how things would go, the worst being that we would lose our flights. And even this wouldn't have been a disaster. We were ready to go the following day, and Luca was in good form. I had a warm meal for him to take with us and a lot of bananas, yoghurt, cheese and some coconut oil as a healthy energy source. Luca was looking forward a lot to Germany. He was hoping to leave his contamination phobia behind him. Could it be that simple? Maybe it was precisely what he needed: a new start.

We settled in quickly in my mother's home. And I had no other choice, as I had to take up my cooking routine as soon as we arrived. Shortly after our journey, Luca got a bad cold. I saw it as a good sign that his body did *not* react with gut symptoms to all this stress. If somebody had asked me before the colitis what I considered Luca's vulnerable spot, I would have said his throat and airways. I had never believed his lower digestive tract to be the weak link in his body. Luca had always been spared when his classmates had been sick with tummy bugs. He had been more susceptible to sore throats and cold symptoms.

Phoenix from the Ashes

"He who heals is right."
(Paracelsus, 1493–1541)

April 2019

For the past 18 months, Luca didn't have any bloody diarrhoea. There were a few days when his gut had felt "different" and had caused him slight pains. Also, his stool had been a bit thinner than usual. We had been concerned that another flare-up could be on the way, but it never happened. However, during these times, Luca showed extra consideration for his gut, took a break from his training for a few days and took it easy. He also didn't eat meat then but poultry and only easy-to-digest vegetable varieties. When Luca wasn't training, he didn't need as much food, which was also easier on his gut. As a preventive measure, he drank several cups of ginger tea daily because of its anti-inflammatory properties. It is possible that on these days, the die-off reactions, as mentioned earlier, were going on in his gut again. But maybe these symptoms were just digestive irregularities, which can occur in everybody's gut. However, because of his medical history, Luca was very alarmed.

During one of these very mild "flares" (if

they could be called this at all), he remarked: "It is strange, really. I just don't know what is going to happen now." – "Yes", I answered, "We don't know. We have to let it happen and stay calm." I realised this was exactly the attitude he had always lacked. His gut forced him to practise equanimity. I also contemplated how his terrible diarrhoea had forced him to let go of everything. During his flares, Luca, the absolute control freak, had not even been able to make it to the toilet and had lost control over everything.

Maybe it was the intelligence of his body-mind-soul-system which had forced him to correct his inner attitude. Perhaps his illness was a means to make him feel that there are life situations beyond our control. Instead of worrying and riding the thought loop carousel again, accepting this fact allows us to take action in areas where we can change something.

On one occasion, Luca had mentioned to me that during his flare-ups, he had not actually felt that bad because, for once, he had been able to give up the constant fight. I remembered an often cited wordplay from the Swiss author Max Frisch which had stayed in my mind since my school days: *"...wir erleben keine [Zufälle], die nicht uns gehören. Am Ende ist es immer das Fällige, was uns zufällt (1)."* Word plays typically don't translate well, but to me, this means that we don't experience coincidences that don't belong to us. Ultimately, what we are receptive to inevitably "falls upon us". Luca's colitis had not happened to him by chance.

We continued our conversation, and Luca noted that it somehow fitted together that he had gotten the colitis. It would always bring him back down to earth and the ground of reality, confronting him with the uncertainty of life. I answered that the "ground of reality" was the same for everybody else. Nobody knew if they would still be healthy in the next year or what the future might hold. The only difference was that most other people were more successful in suppressing these thoughts than he. For this reason, living in the here and now would be all the more important, I added.

"My body is doing what it has to do," Luca stated. "It is cleaning up. After each flare, I was better than before and felt more capable and awake. I also had to eat less afterwards but still had more energy." Luca also told me his contamination phobia had returned a few days ago. Although he had tried to suppress it, it kept haunting him and had stressed him extremely. "Even my eyelids were twitching", he said. "Do you know when I experienced this for the last time? Before the Christmas play at Primary School."

After our conversation, I started making chicken soup for Luca. I noticed that my breathing was very shallow. I had prepared the last "magic chicken soup" before our departure in October 2017. All of a sudden, I was taken back to our dark times. But I told myself that Luca's gut was in a completely different state now than before. He had very mild gut symptoms, and that was all for the moment, nothing less and nothing more. "Faith – hope – confidence. Stay peaceful and at ease," I gently said to myself. I breathed in and out consciously a few times. Then I repeated the mantra "Present moment – only moment" in my head. I had been successful in not letting my thoughts about the past take control. When Luca ate his soup later on, he said: "This is the best soup I have ever eaten."

As time passed, indispositions like this one became rarer and less intense. Instead, Luca had suffered from a few colds since his last flare-up. Some of them were accompanied by fever and vomiting. However, Luca's gut had remained unaffected, and he had not reacted with diarrhoea.

Today Luca weighs 70 kilograms, 14 kilos more than during his worst disease phase. He also has grown a few more centimetres since his diagnosis in 2016. I regard this as a positive sign. With a height of 178 centimetres, he has the ideal body mass index. Luca trains outdoors and in any weather every day. Compared to the Northwest of Ireland, there are a lot of hours of sunshine here in Southern Germany. Sun and light have an enormous impact on Luca's well-being. Sunlight is essential for him, as a sufficient vitamin D level is crucial for an individual with an autoimmune disease.

Besides, Luca's diet, the probiotic bacteria he is ingesting in fermented foods and as a food supplement, and exercising in the open air contribute significantly to his health. Luca's training allows him to be in a state of flow and feel well, balanced and fulfilled. Every day, he feels he is moving closer to his goal, which makes him happy. He is being loved and gets the support he needs to become well and whole again, physically, mentally, emotionally and spiritually.

Luca is grateful that his colitis helped him to find his present diet. He doesn't miss anything, be it grains and the products made thereof, sugar and sweets or processed foods. With his special diet, Luca is symptom-free and feels great while training for several hours daily. That makes a day and night difference to him, who avoided leaving the house for years because he had been afraid of fainting for lack of energy.

I hope that his contamination phobia will also pass by. Luca's brain will become less susceptible to stress when his microbiome is in balance again. And his new experiences, together with the plasticity of his brain, will make it possible for the deep trails his fearful thoughts have left behind in specific brain areas to be overwritten. It will take time, but anything is possible.

It is repeatedly claimed that chronic inflammatory bowel disease cannot be cured. Luckily, what we are experiencing with Luca's colitis is entirely different, and interestingly, holistic therapists don't agree with this dogma either. So where does this limited belief come from, and what if it simply isn't true? How are the terms "curable" or "incurable" defined anyway? Is a person "cured" or "healed" if symptom-free without drugs?

Is it possible that the orthodox medical approach has tremendous shortcomings and, therefore, cannot meet the challenges that chronic conditions such as inflammatory bowel disease pose? And what if the drugs that conventional doctors – in close cooperation with the pharmaceutical industry – employ as weapons against these diseases are not the right tool? Do conventional physicians exhaust all available options to help IBD patients? And if not, is it legitimate to claim that these diseases can't be cured? And is such a statement not merely an expression of capitulation?

As mainstream practitioners have adopted the restrictive belief that there is no cure for IBD, what they offer their patients is limited to prescribing the standard medication.

Do physicians ever think about what it means for their patients to be labelled as "chronically ill", implying that their illness is for life? In this context, the body-mind practitioner Lissa Rankin claims that by giving pessimistic prognoses to their patients, doctors programme negative beliefs into their patients' subconscious minds and provoke stress reactions that are more harmful than helpful to them. *(2)* All of this triggers what is known as the "nocebo-effect", the power of negative thinking. Rankin asks if doctors, crushing all hope for a cure, are not actually paving the way for the fulfilment of their negative prophecies. Although she appreciates her colleagues' wish to be honest with their patients and to respect their patients' responsibility for themselves, she believes it is better to give them hope. Optimism and hope lead to a relaxation response supporting the body's self-repair mechanisms. *(3)*

A trusting relationship between patient and practitioner and a feeling of safety, being cared for and in good hands can also lead to a relaxation response by interrupting a patient's stress reaction. *(4)* Rankin states this is a precondition for the body's self-repair and healing. These findings are by no means new age chatter but scientifically proven facts.

In the past, caring for the patient's emotional well-being was considered a primary task of a doctor. Accordingly, the German physician Dr Kurt Pollak wrote in 1958: "Fear and hopelessness are a bigger hindrance to healing than adverse external conditions. Therefore, the patient shall receive confidence and hope from the words, countenance and gestures of the doctor and the nursing staff. A doctor has to be an optimist by nature. Even in seemingly hopeless cases, he must think: Maybe everything will be well in the end! He may not weaken in his efforts until death has occurred. Again and again, there are unexpected turns which even an experienced doctor would not have thought possible. Above all, the sick person wants to feel that both doctor and nursing staff have time and patience for them and that they address their ailments. More important than verbal promises is a certain confident demeanour of the carer or the physician *(5)*."

When Luca received his colitis diagnosis at age 16 – not even from his gastroenterologist but from a nurse – he was handed a few pills, a prescription and the information brochures of a pharmaceutical company. One of the leaflets gave nutritional advice, including precisely those foods we eliminated from Luca's diet shortly afterwards. One-third of his food was supposed to consist of grains. The recommendation also included a lot of milk and milk products. There was no talk of eliminating sugar, which is highly inflammatory. And for the evenings, a cup of hot chocolate and a serving of milk rice were on the menu. It was pointed out to the patients that a balanced diet was necessary for them. In general, however, they would know best what they could tolerate and which foods to avoid.

At the beginning of my book, I talked about another IBD brochure that filled me with fear and terror; you probably remember. Today, I view its content even more critically. Genetics ranked first as a possible cause of the disease, whereas lifestyle factors were not mentioned at all. Patients were familiarized with all conventional IBD medications, from possibly relatively mild drugs to immunosuppressants and biologicals and their most common side effects. Sadly, the reality of most patients is such that they gradually need more potent drugs, which mostly also have more severe adverse effects.

The brochure acquainted patients with their possible "fate", the surgical removal of their colon. It was also pointed out that IBD patients have a higher cancer risk. What was not mentioned, of course, is that this can also be due to medications that suppress the immune system and a failure to address the underlying root causes of the disease.

I would like to know why severely ill people are immediately confronted with the worst-case scenario, the surgical removal of their colon, when it should be the highest goal of a doctor to avoid this. Have the providers of this "helpful information for patients" ever heard of empathy or psychology? Or could this be an attempt to deliberately intimidate patients known to be at risk of developing a new flare-up when under severe stress?

Our experiences on the day of Luca's diagnosis and after it don't cast a positive light on the conventional medical system. Do representatives of mainstream medicine nowadays really haven't got more to offer to their patients than handing them information from the pharmaceutical industry and thus triggering the nocebo effect? Is this a good way to tell their patients that they suffer from a disease which allegedly will affect them for the rest of their lives?

Luca and I have developed our own positive understanding of colitis: Luca's body-mind-soul-system imposes certain conditions on him, and if he responds to them, he is rewarded with a lot of energy, vitality, and mental clarity. These conditions are probably linked to his genetics and may apply to him for his entire life. Meeting these conditions implies a special diet and a particular lifestyle. What this means is that he is living according to his very own personal needs. This self-image fundamentally differs from believing you have a lifelong chronic and incurable disease.

For patients who are convinced that their chronic inflammatory bowel disease is not curable, it is consequently not possible to say that they *had* ulcerative colitis or Crohn's disease. Instead, the phrase: "I *have* ulcerative colitis, or I *have* Crohn's disease" is imprinted in their consciousness – and maybe even worse, in their subconsciousness – for the rest of their lives. That hugely impacts their psyche as you can only become healthy if you can let go of an illness and put it behind you.

Luca and I are always talking about his illness in the past tense. Of course, we cannot rule out that another flare-up may occur sometime. Nobody can know this. However, we are convinced that Luca's gut is not the same as it had been at his diagnosis. For the past years, Luca's microbiome, and with it his immune system, have continuously developed in a healthier direction.

On top of this, his digestive system doesn't have to deal with foods it can't tolerate anymore. So Luca's gut has no more reason to be inflamed. A colonoscopy, with which I don't want to burden Luca yet, will show us at some point in the future what it looks like in his gut and if we are right. (Although this is not about being right! We are just so grateful that Luca is well.) Luca feels that his gut is robust and resilient again. His symptoms have disappeared, but the fear of a possible relapse, which the doctors and the pharmaceutical industry also fuel, is still present. Even today, he is still checking his stools for any traces of blood.

Also, Luca's facial skin is returning to normal. And the skin is known to be not only the mirror of the soul but also that of gut health.

Luca and I had been back to my old home town for a good while when I bumped into a former school friend. It must have been about 35 years ago since we last met. We said hello and started talking. After a short time, we discovered that we both had a son with ulcerative colitis. What a strange coincidence.

I told her about our healing success with the SCD and the GAPS diet. She said that her son didn't want to hear anything about diets. When his disease symptoms occurred for the first time before his leaving cert, this turned all his plans for the future upside down. However, he succeeded in his dream job. Nobody was supposed to know about his condition because this might be the end of his career.

She said that he was relying entirely on his medication and that he was on immunosuppressants. When he had moved from home a few years ago, he had to promise his gastroenterologist that he would keep away from certain drugs if one of his colleagues should intend to prescribe them to him. These medications would be too dangerous for a young patient like him who still had all his life ahead of him. Nobody would be able to predict their effects.

I was shocked to hear that. After our conversation, both of us continued with our shopping. I bought some organic, unpasteurised sauerkraut for Luca. That represented one of his remedies.

The conversation with my former schoolmate followed me for a long time. Every patient must find a way of handling the disease. We have found a path that is appropriate for Luca. I am curious about where his journey will lead him.

APPENDIX

Further Information on the Blood Group Diet

The blood group diet is based on Dr d'Adamo's hypothesis that there is a correlation between a person's blood group and their ability to tolerate certain foods. D'Adamo believes that the various blood groups developed in different phases of human evolution. He is convinced that each blood group carries the genetic message of our forefathers' dietary habits and behaviours. Our immune and digestive systems still have an affinity to the foods that our ancestors with the same blood type used to eat, so Dr d'Adamo.

He states blood type 0 is the eldest, followed by blood types A and B, and then blood type AB, which is the rarest. In Germany, 38 to 40 per cent of the total population have blood type 0. This blood type is supposed to have developed about 40 000 BC when our forefathers were still hunters and gatherers. Their primary energy source consisted of animal protein, as they ate a lot of meat. According to Dr d'Adamo, individuals with this blood type have a very active immune system that reacts promptly and is highly sensitive to new influences and changes.

In Dr d'Adamo's view, individuals who, based on their blood type, belong to the group of hunters and gatherers can tolerate meat very well and even need meat. However, their metabolisms have difficulty coping with grains (especially wheat) and milk. That is because, from an evolutionary point of view, the digestive tract of humans was confronted with these foods much later and is, therefore, not genetically programmed to digest them. Gluten tends to irritate the small intestine of persons with blood type 0 in particular and should thus be eliminated from their diets, says Dr d'Adamo.

Acknowledgements

I want to express my deep appreciation to everybody who is prepared to go the extra mile. Thanks to everyone who supported me directly or indirectly in creating this book.

Thank you to the brilliant Functional Medicine practitioners who generously share their insights and experience on the internet or in the form of books so that we can all learn from them.

I thank my friend and colleague Uta Haas for her support and friendship. Thank you to Diane Roemer for her linguistic suggestions as an American native speaker.

I also thank Catherina Dilworth, who probably isn't aware of how much she helped me when I couldn't see the light at the end of the tunnel. A big thank you to Dr Eric Dilworth for proofreading and his appreciation of my work.

I am grateful to my mother, whose love and support I can always be sure of, even if I may not always make it easy for her.

I give special thanks to my inner pilot light. And, of course, to my partner and our son. Thank you so much for your love and for being there. Without your support and patience, I would never have found the time to write this book.

Notes

All quotations originating from sources in German have been translated by the author into English. If the sources are books of which also English editions exist, the author's translations can differ. However, this should not affect the content.

All internet sources have been looked up for the last time between the 17th and the 18th of April 2021.

Background

(1) https://www.cdc.gov/ibd/features/IBD-more-chronic-diseases.html
(2) https://www.stvincents.ie/crohns-colitis-and-covid-19-latest-research/

Chapter 1

(1) Chris Kresser, Unconventional Medicine Join the Revolution to Reinvent Healthcare, Reverse Chronic Disease and Create a Practice You Love, Lioncrest, Austin, 2017, p. 62.
(2) Dr Tom O'Bryan, The Autoimmune Fix, Rodale Inc., New York, 2016, p. 136 f.
(3) Dr med William Davis, Weizenwampe: Warum Weizen dick und krank macht, dt. Erstausgabe, Goldmann Verlag, München, 2013, p. 128.

Chapter 3

(1) Raman Prasad, Colitis & Me: A Story of
Recovery, Published by SCD Recipe LLC, First
Printing 2003, p. 6.

Chapter 6

(1)
https://www.barmer.de/blob/71456/1f5b78999d9
b260f1b2a6ccbc4518170/data/die-chronisch-
entzuendlichen-darmerkrankungen-morbus-crohn-
und-colitus-ulcerosa.pdf.

Chapter 7

(1) "Gut and Psychology Syndrome", N. Campbell-
McBride, MD,
http://orthomolecular.org/library/jom/2008/pdf/
2008-v23n02-p090.pdf.
(2) Seattle Children's Hospital. "Novel diet therapy
helps children with crohn's disease and ulcerative
colitis reach remission." ScienceDaily. ScienceDaily,
28 December 2016.
<www.sciencedaily.com/releases/2016/12/161228
171130.htm>.
(3) Lissa Rankin, Warum Gedanken stärker sind als
Medizin: Wissenschaftliche Beweise für die
Selbstheilungskraft, Kösel Verlag, Verlagsgruppe

Random House, München, 3. Aufl., 2017, p. 37.

(4) Eckart von Hirschhausen, Wunder wirken Wunder, Rowohlt Taschenbuch Verlag, Hamburg, 2018, p. 185.

(5) https://www.jillcarnahan.com/2016/08/21/power-subconscious-mind-heal/.

(6) "Zonulin and Its Regulation of Intestinal Barrier Function: The Biological Door to Inflammation, Autoimmunity, and Cancer." Alessio Fasano, 01. Jan. 2011, https://journals.physiology.org/doi/full/10.1152/physrev.00003.2008.

(7) https://chriskresser.com/pioneering-researcher-alessio-fasano-m-d-on-gluten-autoimmunity-leaky-gut/

(8) Irish Independent.ie dated 20.2.2017 "Irish man (30) cycled 27,369 km of this planet in spite of debilitating bowel disease. "

Chapter 8

(1) Sabine Wery von Limont, Das geheime Leben der Seele, Mosaik Verlag, München, 2018, p. 251/252.

(2) https://chriskresser.com/what-everybody-ought-to-know-but-doesnt-about-heartburn-gerd/.

(3) Deepak Chopra, Reinventing the Body, Resurrecting the Soul, 2009 by Rider, an imprint of Ebury Publishing.

(4) Ornish, D., et al., Changes in prostate gene expression in men undergoing an intensive nutrition and lifestyle intervention, PNAS 2008, vol. 105, no. 24: 8369-8374.
(5) Bruce Lipton, Biology of Belief, 10th Anniversary Edition, Hay House Inc., Carlsbad, USA, 2015, p. 48/49.
(6) Dr. Antje R. Weseler, „Über den Genen: Epigenetik – Teil 1",
https://www.researchgate.net/publication/2582183 68_Uber_den_Genen_Epigenetik_-_Teil_1.
(7) http://old.theDrcom/betrayal-docuseries/.
(8) http://old.theDrcom/betrayal-docuseries/.
(9) Fei Ke, Praveen Kumar Yadav, and Liu Zhan Ju, "Herbal Medicine in the Treatment of Ulcerative Colitis", Saudi J Gastroenterol. 2012 Jan-Feb, 18 (1): 3-10. doi: 10.4103/1319-3767.91726,
https://www.ncbi.nlm.nih.gov/pmc/articles/PMC 3271691/.
(10) Richard N. Fedorak, MD, FRCPC, "Probiotics in the Management of Ulcerative Colitis", Gastroenterol Hepatol (N Y). 2010 Nov; 6 (11): 688-690. PMC 3033537,
https://www.ncbi.nlm.nih.gov/pmc/articles/PMC 3033537/.
(11) Prof Dr M. Axt-Gadermann, Schlau mit Darm, Südwest Verlag, München, 2. Auflage, 2017, p. 94.
(12) Prof Dr M. Axt-Gadermann, Schön mit Darm,

Südwest Verlag, München, 2017, p. 130.

Chapter 9

(1) Pentasa: Uses, Dosage & Side Effects,
https://www.drugs.com/drug-class/5-
aminosalicylates.html#.
(2) https://www.prnewswire.com/news-
releases/the-global-inflammatory-bowel-diseases-
ibd-drug-market-is-estimated-at-6-7bn-in-2017-and-
7-6bn-in-2023--300688523.html.
https://www.reportlinker.com/p04890882
(3) https://www.drugs.com/sfx/pentasa-side-
effects.html.
(4) Uwe Karstädt, Entgiften statt Vergiften, TAS
Distribution Ltd., London, 2007.
(5) www.amymyersmd.com/2018/08/l-glutamine-
repairing-leaky-gut.

Chapter 10

(1) Prof Dr Michaela Axt-Gadermann, Schön mit
Darm, Südwest Verlag, München, 2017, p. 107.
(2) Prof Dr Michaela Axt-Gadermann, Schön mit
Darm, Südwest Verlag, München, 2017, p. 115.
(3) Dr Natasha Campbell-McBride, Gut and
Psychology Syndrome, Medinform Publishing, UK,
2016, p. 123.
(4) Sarah Ballantyne PhD, The Paleo Approach,
Victory Belt Publishing Inc., Las Vegas, USA, 2013,

p. 148.
(5) Prof Dr Dr Kurt S. Zänker, Das Immunsystem des Menschen: Bindeglied zwischen Körper und Seele. Originalsausgabe – München: Verlag C. H. Beck, 1996, p. 117/118.
(6) Jesper Juul, Dein kompetentens Kind, Rowohlt Taschenbuch Verlag, Hamburg, 2009, p. 85.

Chapter 11

(1) Bruce Lipton, Biology of Belief, 10th Anniversary Edition, Hay House Inc., Carlsbad, USA, 2015, p. 94/95.
(2) Bruce Lipton, Biology of Belief, 10th Anniversary Edition, Hay House Inc., Carlsbad, USA, 2015, p. 132.
(3) Eckart von Hirschhausen, Wunder wirken Wunder, Rowohlt Taschenbuch Verlag, Hamburg, 2018, p. 54.
(4) Bruce Lipton, Biology of Belief, 10th Anniversary Edition, Hay House Inc., Carlsbad, USA, 2015, p. 138.

Chapter 12

(1) Monika Holthoff-Stenger, „Meuternde Mikroben", natur. Das Magazin für Natur, Umwelt und besseres Leben, Ausgabe 10/15, p. 94–96.
(2) G. Moser, „Bedeutung von Stress und Depression bei chronisch-entzündlichen

Darmerkrankungen", Journal für
Gastroenterologische und Hepatologische
Erkrankungen, 2005; 3 (2), 26–30.
(3) Daniel Goleman, Emotionale Intelligenz,
Deutscher Taschenbuchverlag, München,
Jubiläumsedition 2014, p. 273 f.
(4) Daniel Goleman, Emotionale Intelligenz,
Deutscher Taschenbuchverlag, München,
Jubiläumsedition 2014, p. 274.
(5) Daniel Goleman, Emotionale Intelligenz,
Deutscher Taschenbuchverlag, München,
Jubiläumsedition 2014, p. 273.
(6) Sabine Wery von Limont, Das geheime Leben
der Seele, Mosaik Verlag, München, 2018, p. 54.

Chapter 13

(1) Max Frisch, Tagebuch, 1946–1949, Suhrkamp,
Frankfurt/M., 1950, p. 463–464.
(2) Lisa Rankin, Warum Gedanken stärker sind als
Medizin: Wissenschaftliche Beweise für die
Selbstheilungskraft, Kösel Verlag, Verlagsgruppe
Random House, München, 3. Aufl., 2017, p. 75.
(3) Lisa Rankin, Warum Gedanken stärker sind als
Medizin: Wissenschaftliche Beweise für die
Selbstheilungskraft, Kösel Verlag, Verlagsgruppe
Random House, München, 3. Aufl., 2017, p. 75.
(4) Lisa Rankin, Warum Gedanken stärker sind als
Medizin: Wissenschaftliche Beweise für die
Selbstheilungskraft, Kösel Verlag, Verlagsgruppe

Random House, München, 3. Aufl., 2017, p. 89.
(5) Dr Kurt Pollak, Das ärztliche Hausbuch. Ein praktischer Ratgeber für die Familie, Bertelsmann Verlag, Gütersloh, 1958, 1965, p. 78.

**More about
The Gut Flora**

(1) Dr Natasha Campbell-McBride, Gut and Psychology Syndrome, Medinform Publishing, UK, 2016, p. 17.

Bibliography

Prof Dr Michaela Axt-Gadermann, Schlau mit Darm, Südwest Verlag, München, 2. Aufl., 2017.

Prof Dr Michaela Axt-Gadermann, Schön mit Darm, Südwest Verlag, München, 2017.

Sarah Ballantyne PhD, The Paleo Approach, Victory Belt Publishing Inc., Las Vegas, USA, 2013.

Dieter Beck, Krankheit als Selbstheilung: Wie körperliche Krankheiten ein Versuch zur seelischen Heilung sein können, Suhrkamp Taschenbuchverlag, Frankfurt, 1985.

Jörg Blech, Gene sind kein Schicksal. Wie wir unsere Erbanlagen und unser Leben steuern können, Fischer Verlag, Frankfurt, 2012.

Dr med Max Otto Bruker, Unsere Nahrung – unser Schicksal, 43. Auflage 2009, c Emu-Verlags Gmbh, Lahnstein, Erstausgabe 1969 unter dem Titel „Schicksal aus der Küche".

Dr Natasha Campbell-McBride, Gut and Psychology Syndrome, Medinform Publishing, UK, 2016.

Deepak Chopra, Reinventing the Body, Resurrecting the Soul, Rider, an imprint of Ebury Publishing, 2009.

Dr Peter J. D'Adamo, The GenoType Diet: Change Your Genetic Destiny to live the longest, fullest and healthiest Life possible, Harmony, 2007.

Dr med William Davis, Weizenwampe: Warum Weizen dick und krank macht, dt. Erstausgabe, Goldmann Verlag, München, 2013.

Larry Dossey, Heilungsfelder: Wenn die Seele den Körper heilt. Psychoneuroimmunologie, dt. Erstausgabe, Crotona Verlag, Amerang, 2012.

Gulia Enders, Darm mit Charme, Ullstein Buchverlage, Berlin, 2014.

Prof Dr Alessio Fasano, Susie Flaherty, Die ganze Wahrheit über Gluten, Südwest Verlag, München, 2015.

Daniel Goleman, Emotionale Intelligenz, Jubiläumsedition, Deutscher Taschenbuchverlag, München, 2014.

Elaine Gottschall, Breaking the Vicious Cycle: Intestinal Health through Diet, Kirkton Press Ltd, Ontario, Canada, Fifteenth Printing, 2014.

Hans-Ulrich Grimm, Die Ernährungslüge: Wie uns die Lebensmittelindustrie um den Verstand bringt, Drömer Verlag, München, 2003.

Mimi Guarneri, MD, 108 Pearls to Awaken Your Healing Potential, Hay House Inc., Carlsbad, USA, 2017.

John Harrison, M.D., Love Your Disease, It's keeping You Healthy!, Peacock Books, 2018.

Prof Dr med Wilhelm Heupke, Wisse – Erkenne – Handle. Ein Volksbuch der Gesundheitspflege, Wiesbadener Buchgesellschaft, Wiesbaden, 1960.

Eckart von Hirschhausen, Wunder wirken Wunder, Rowohlt Taschenbuch Verlag, Hamburg, 2018.

Bernd Hontschik, Körper, Seele, Mensch – Versuch über die Kunst des Heilens, Suhrkamp Verlag, Frankfurt, 2006.

Jesper Juul, Dein kompetentens Kind, Rowohlt Taschenbuch Verlag, Hamburg, 2009.

Uwe Karstädt, Entgiften statt Vergiften, TAS Distribution Ltd., London, 2007.

Dr. Norbert Kriegisch, Ich fühle mich krank –

warum findet niemand etwas?, Scorpio Verlag, München, 2018.

Bruce Lipton, Biology of Belief, 10th Anniversary Edition, Hay House Inc., Carlsbad, USA, 2015.

Dr Alex Loyd, Dr Ben Johnson, Der Healing Code, Deutsche Erstausgabe, Rowohlt Taschenbuch Verlag, 2012.

Dr med Roy Martina, Emotionale Balance, Deutsche Ausgabe, KOHA-Verlag, Burgrain, 3. Aufl.

Dr Joseph Mercola, Fat for Fuel, Hay House Inc., Carlsbad, USA, 2017.

Dr Amy Myers, Die Autoimmun-Lösung: Ein gesundes Immunsystem beginnt im Darm, Irisiana Verlag, München, 2016.

Dr Amy Myers: Die Autoimmunlösung: Das Kochbuch, Irisiana Verlag, München, 2019.

Dr Tom O'Bryan, The Autoimmune Fix, Rodale Inc., New York, 2016.

Candace B. Pert, PhD, Molecules of Emotion, Simon & Schuster, London, 1998.

Dr Kurt Pollak, Das ärztliche Hausbuch. Ein praktischer Ratgeber für die Familie, Bertelsmann Verlag, Gütersloh, 1958, 1965

Raman Prasad, Colitis & Me: A Story of Recovery, Published by SCD Recipe LLC, First Printing 2003.

Raman Prasad, Recipes for the Specific Carbohydrate Diet (With a foreword by Raquel Nieves, M. D.), Fair Winds Press, USA, 2008.

Lisa Rankin, Warum Gedanken stärker sind als Medizin: Wissenschaftliche Beweise für die Selbstheilungskraft, Kösel Verlag, Verlagsgruppe Random House, München, 3. Aufl., 2017.

Dr Joan I. Rosenberg, 90 Seconds to a Life You Love, Yellow Kite, GB, 2019.

Dr Klaus Dietrich Runow, Der Darm denkt mit: Wie Bakterien, Pilze und Allergien das Nervensystem beeinflussen, Südwest Verlag, München, 2011.

Dr rer nat C. Schmincke, Chinesische Medizin für die westliche Welt, 3. aktualisierte Auflage, Springer Medizin Verlag, Heidelberg 2004 und 2007.

David Servan-Schreiber, Das Antikrebs-Buch, Taschenbuchausgabe, Goldmann Verlag, München,

2010.

Katharina Sonnleitner, Reiner Schmid, Der Darm –
Zentrum der Gesundheit, 2. Aufl., Verlag
Ernährung und Gesundheit, Inning am Ammersee,
2010.

Cornelia Stolze, Krank durch Medikamente: Wenn
Antibiotika depressiv, Schlafmittel dement und
Blutdrucksenker impotent machen, Piper Verlag,
München, 2014.

Sabine Wery von Limont, Das geheime Leben der
Seele, Mosaik Verlag, München, 2018.

Peter Yoda, Ein Medizinischer Insider packt aus,
Sensei Verlag, Kernen, 2007.

Prof Dr Dr Kurt S. Zänker, Das Immunsystem des
Menschen: Bindeglied zwischen Körper und Seele,
Originalausgabe, Verlag C. H. Beck, München,
1996.

Websites

In English:
https://www.mygutsense.com
https://www.nimbal.org
https://www.chriskresser.com
https://www.zachbushmd.com
https://geneticliteracyproject.org/2017/08/24/gmos-revealed-documentary-series-delivers-familiar-arguments-fringe/
https://www.gmosrevealed.com/
https://www.scdrecipe.com (Raman Prasad's website)
https://www.dietagainstdisease.com/
https://www.autoimmunesummit.com
https://www.theglutensummit.com
https://www.youtube.com/watch?v=IKQgLf0b_uI (Dr. Joel Wallach, "Cereal Killers: Danger of Wheat, Gluten & Grains", Youngevity Classic Lecture)
https://www.doctormurray.com (Digestive Health Summit)
https://www.drjockers.com/10-ways-improve-stomach-acid-levels
https://www.clinicaleducation.org

In German:
https://scd-blog.de (Aleksandra Hadzik and I are publishing together on this website.)
https://autoimmunportal.de

https://zentrum-der-gesundheit.de
https://haus-des-heilens.news
https://online-kongresse.info/events/morbus-crohn-und-colitis-ulcerosa-online-kongress/
https://online-kongresse.info/events/autoimmun-online-kongress/

For Your Personal Notes...

For Your Personal Notes...

For Your Personal Notes...

259